LOVE, INTIMACY AND ONLINE DATING

Love, Intimacy and Online Dating: How a Global Pandemic Redefined Romantic Relationships is an innovative work that explores the concept of intimacy during the COVID-19 pandemic. The book provides an overview of the online dating world and apps, the use of which gradually became common as the pandemic restricted people's interaction in the physical world. The author's extensive research conducted during the pandemic posits a comprehensive understanding of the individual's motivation to join a dating app and explores its varied aspects.

This thoroughly researched book explores the themes and elements of online dating and examines the users' motivation for joining a dating app, for seeking intimacy as well as for self-presentation on the app. Portolan examines the underlying politics and role of infrastructure of dating apps and describes how gender, power and intimacy intersect to create new intimacy phenomena. She also utilises her research to put forth the key concept of 'Jagged Love', which describes a user's cyclical relationship with dating apps during the pandemic, and the gap between a user's act to seek familiar romantic narratives and the app's inability to deliver against these ideas. The chapters further explore the differences between virtual and In Real Life (IRL) intimacy, the generation of gender and the emanation of stereotypical cultural ideals that the users sought through the apps. The book serves as an invaluable discussion on the pandemic's impact on modifying the definitions of romance and intimacy.

This book will be useful for highlighting the impact social factors can have on familiar concepts and the effects of the COVID-19 pandemic on the definition of love and intimacy, making it fascinating for students, academics and professionals interested in relationships, digital media and gender. It will also be useful in enhancing the comprehension of love and romance in the fields of social science.

Lisa Portolan is a researcher and author from Sydney, Australia. Her research focusses on intimacy, romance, dating apps and gender, and she regularly writes for publications like *The Conversation.* She is the author of best-selling titles and is often featured on programmes, such as *the Today Show*, *the Drum* and beyond, while her top ten podcast, *Slow Love*, documented dating and love during the pandemic.

LOVE, INTIMACY AND ONLINE DATING

How a Global Pandemic Redefined Romantic Relationships

Lisa Portolan

Routledge
Taylor & Francis Group
LONDON AND NEW YORK

Cover image: © Getty Images

First published 2023
by Routledge
4 Park Square, Milton Park, Abingdon, Oxon OX14 4RN

and by Routledge
605 Third Avenue, New York, NY 10158

Routledge is an imprint of the Taylor & Francis Group, an informa business

British Library Cataloguing-in-Publication Data
A catalogue record for this book is available from the British Library

Library of Congress Cataloging-in-Publication Data
Names: Portolan, Lisa, author.
Title: Love, intimacy and online dating : how a global pandemic redefined romantic relationships / Lisa Portolan.
Description: Abingdon, Oxon ; New York, NY : Routledge, 2023. |
Includes bibliographical references and index. |
Identifiers: LCCN 2022027341 (print) | LCCN 2022027342 (ebook) |
ISBN 9780367637040 (hardback) | ISBN 9780367637033 (paperback) |
ISBN 9781003120353 (ebook)
Subjects: LCSH: Dating (Social customs) | Intimacy (Psychology) |
Interpersonal relations. | COVID-19 Pandemic, 2020—Social aspects.
Classification: LCC HQ801 .P86 2023 (print) | LCC HQ801 (ebook) |
DDC 306.73—dc23/eng/20220627
LC record available at https://lccn.loc.gov/2022027341
LC ebook record available at https://lccn.loc.gov/2022027342

ISBN: 9780367637040 (hbk)
ISBN: 9780367637033 (pbk)
ISBN: 9781003120353 (ebk)

DOI: 10.4324/9781003120353

Typeset in Bembo
by codeMantra

CONTENTS

1 Introduction 1

2 Social context 8

3 Jagged Love – The conflict: Romance vs dating apps 20

4 (Digital) intimacy vs IRL intimacy and why the distinction *still* needs to be made 38

5 High-Maintenance Girls and Aussie Blokes: Love and gender stereotypes during Covid times 51

6 Messiness – Three anecdotes 69

References *91*
Index *105*

1

INTRODUCTION

From a young age I was intrigued by the idea of love. As a child, I was introverted and strange. I buried myself in literature: the Bronte sisters, Shelley, Keats, Duras and a good measure of Shakespeare. The type of white, western education, that nobody really wants much of these days. And alongside that, I imbibed a heavy dose of rom-coms. I was the last child, with two older sisters. There was a significant age gap between us – which meant I ended up watching cult eighties films at a very young age. Movies like *The Breakfast Club*, *Pretty in Pink*, *Sixteen Candles*, and later, *Pretty Woman* and *Only You*. It might have been this acute recipe of narrativised love that resulted in me being an overly romantic teenager. I was consumed by the idea of finding 'the one' and was quite sure that my life hadn't started until that milestone had been achieved. In my twenties, and long before the time dating apps and online dating was conceptualised, I threw myself into the intimacy maelstrom with the type of passion only an idealist can summon. But as the years passed me by, and I accrued a series of broken, damaged and unsuccessful relationships, the utopia of love started to lose a sense of practical potential. It occurred to me that the type of love that swept you away was reserved for the realm of literature and movies, or indeed, the imagination. Spaces which were highly fictionalised, orchestrated and yes, imagined. Locations where the perfunctory and often awkward elements of real bodies didn't exist.

However, despite this pragmatic view on relationships, my fixation with the idea of love, romance and all things intimate continued. In my late thirties, while working at one of these incredibly cool PR agencies with in-house table tennis tournaments, video games and an open bar, I found myself seated in an open-floor format, where non-work conversations consistently revolved around one topic – the interpretation of discussions, images and potential matches on dating apps. Having never used a dating app myself, these exchanges piqued my interest.

DOI: 10.4324/9781003120353-1

Many of my colleagues were in their early twenties, and had never known a world sans dating apps – and while this didn't seem of particular relevance to them, I couldn't help but wonder, how did dating apps change intimacy? As intimacies (hook-ups, dates and romantic relationships) were filtered through the dating app architecture and infrastructure, what types of new intimacies were produced? Were gender stereotypes and scripts reinforced or subverted as a result of dating apps? And how did dating apps change or continue the milestones expected in romantic narratives?

The fieldwork conducted as part of my research occurred from March to June 2020, which coincided with the first COVID-19 lockdown in NSW – this also turned out to be unprecedented dating territory. With physical distancing orders in place, and most people either working or studying from home, dating apps became the key (if only) conduit for relationships. Dating apps across the world reported immense surges in sign-ups and use. This wasn't in and of itself revolutionary – with face-to-face meetings no longer possible, it was reasonable to imagine that the majority of singles or non-singles would turn towards dating apps to seek an intimate other. Alongside this, meeting an intimate other became increasingly important, as singles faced the reality of lock-down, alone. In a time of uncertainty, the desire for certainty, tradition and the known became paramount. Enter the romantic masterplot(s). What is the romantic masterplot(s)? Well, it's only one of the most widely understood narratives in white, western society, and it surfaced in a myriad of ways in my research. The reason I use the term masterplot(s) is because the idea of a single romantic masterplot reduces the sometimes complex and contradictory messaging and narratives associated with romance. As recent work by Radway indicates, the narratives and thematics within masterplot(s) are often incorporated, subverted or changed in many different ways – as will later be explored. How did these masterplot(s) interact with the digital landscape, and in particular, dating apps?

Whilst scholars such as Hobbs, Owen and Gerber (2016) argue that:

> A 'digital revolution' is underway with regard to dating, courtship and modern romance. Unlike previous generations, single adults today, particularly those living in large metropolitan centres, have a seemingly endless variety of potential romantic and sexual partners available through the social networks and algorithms of their smartphones.

I would contend that this digital revolution in the ambit of love and hook-ups was well underway prior to the COVID-19 lockdown. Whilst the pandemic might have accelerated the episodic use of dating apps, they were already one of the main sources of relationship facilitation. Over the past two decades, dating apps have become a central point of discussion in relation to dating, relationships and intimacy. Many Australian singles (and non-singles) frequently use an app or multiple apps to navigate and negotiate relationships (Bailey, 2012). Independent research indicates that rates of dating app usage have seen significant growth in Australia across the last decade (YouGov, 2017). A survey of 2000 people conducted by Nielsen in 2010 revealed that 25 percent of Australians had tried dating apps (Bailey, 2012). In 2015, Tinder announced that 15 percent of the Australian population had joined the app (Bruce-Smith, 2017). Most recently, a 2017 study conducted by YouGov indicated that 52 percent of Australian singles had used a dating app to make a romantic connection. The same study indicated that usage was particularly high for single Australians between 25 and 34, with 60 percent having used a dating app to make a romantic connection.

Opinions relating to dating app usage in contemporary media have varied; however, an overarching narrative has emerged, in which dating apps have colonised love, created a virtual emotional marketplace, fostered a hook-up culture and devalued traditional institutions such as marriage, monogamy and long-term partnerships. Other negative commentary has centred around health and concern over physical and emotional safety, as well as a perceived rise in Sexually Transmitted Diseases (STDs) as a result of an app-facilitated hook-up culture (AFP, 2019). For older generations who may never have used dating apps (or are suddenly required to take a foray into this space), the censure of the dating app landscape is high, while for younger generations (particularly those within an 18–28-year-old bracket) dating apps present as a pre-condition to romance, an integral part of the dating experience. This younger generation has never dated within an IRL (In Real Life) environment, and many would prefer not to (Fetters, 2018).

In the 2020s, it is hard to imagine a world without dating apps or digitally facilitated relationships. Looking back, computer-based match-making technology had its naissance in the 1960s, but its genealogy can be traced to personal ads in the seventeenth century (Macleod & McArthur, 2018). Brainz (2011) cites the first online dating site as kiss.com, which was registered in 1994, and the mid-nineties saw a rise in similar match-making websites like match.com, RSVP.com and e-harmony. The growth of relationship websites – and, subsequently, mobile dating apps – has been steady across the last 20 years. The last decade saw a panoply of dating apps mushroom, catering towards a diversity of groups and people. The shift to mobile dating app usage significantly changed the dynamic, and its affordances made online dating ubiquitous. Users can now access matches from any location and can also locate matches in situ (for example, by opening Tinder in a bar, users are able to see which singles are closest to them, based on the geo-spatial functionalities).

Leading the dating app charge was Grindr, a geosocial and networking dating app released in 2009, which is available on Android and iOS and can be downloaded from the app store. Tinder was released in 2011, and less than three years later (2014), the platform had registered over one billion users (Rao, 2011). Since then, a proliferation of dating apps has flooded the market (Hinge, Scruff, Happn, Coffee meets Bagel, Bumble, etc.), tailored to different segments of the community. But dating apps are now mainstream. Today, the notion of love, relationships, hook-ups and dating are deeply entangled with dating apps. However, it is undoubtable that the digital world reconfigures 'everyday life' – particularly within the intimacy domain. Ling details this 'everydayness' in relation to texting and mobile phones, writing, 'Nobody sits at home anymore waiting for the phone to ring', and indeed, this Uber-planned approached to the digital and dating is continued within the app environment. What are the limitations of this hyper-coordinateness, and how did COVID, in particular, impact this?

And whilst we would all like to condemn the digital domain as the genesis for the shallowness of the dating environment, there is little analysis of the deep continuities in love and intimacy which dating apps produce and facilitate. While dating apps present as a rupture in the way relationships are instigated and developed – that is, a movement from a physical environment to a digital landscape – they also present a *continuity* in pre-existing relationship dynamics and romantic masterplot(s). As my research demonstrated, despite the 'hook-up' dynamic generated by app architecture like Tinder, users continue to seek to emplot themselves in a romantic narrative.

As a snapshot of my work, I conducted iterative focus groups to gather shared understandings of dating apps but also to shake out any new and different ideas or ways of thinking about dating apps. The focus groups were conducted in Sydney city, and regional participants were provided the option of connecting via Zoom as a result of COVID-19. Participants were asked set questions in the first focus group about their dating app experience, usage practices, personal presentation on app, expectations, and desires. Questions were tailored for the second focus group around trends that emerged, and participants were also asked to design their ideal dating app architecture and functionalities in groups. In-depth interviews were conducted over Zoom and were approximately an hour in length, following a semi-structured format. Eight participants also journaled their experience during the month of March and were asked to do so for at least one hour per week, capturing screen grabs of their experience if they desired.

Twenty participants were recruited: twelve were heterosexual women, six were heterosexual men and two were queer men. Two participants were consensually non-monogamous, the rest were 'single' or were in the preliminary stages of dating ('talking to') someone. The research intended on capturing heterosexual dating app practices, although it did not seek to exclude other sexualities or ways of being.

McAlister argues there is a clear heteronormativity in the romance masterplot (noting here, intentionally singular) and its milestones (for example, first date, moving in, marriage, conceiving a bay, etc.), including its impetus towards the couple norm. The effect of this has been grappled with at length in queer theory, in particular through Tom Boellstorff's (2007, p. 228) theorisation of 'straight time': an epically salient, socially efficacious, and experientially real cultural construction of temporality across a wide range of political and social positions, shaped by and linked to discourses of heteronormativity, capitalism, and modernity. Questions of straight time were particularly interrogated during the debates over the legalisation of same-sex marriage, because – very broadly speaking – marriage is a clear marker in a narrative governed by straight time. As Boellstorff (2007) notes, there was significant tension between the desire of equal rights (i.e. the right to marry) and the desire to resist the imposition of a heteropatriarchal temporal narrative. There are not enough LGBTQ+ participants in my sample for us to make any substantive claims about how app users belonging to these communities interact with the romance masterplot and how any resistance to 'straight time' might complicate this.

Notably, questions of gender are fundamental to dating apps. They are foundational to app algorithms, as this is the key way in which a user indicates their preference as to whose profiles the app will show them. There have been several studies examining apps through the lens of gender. Caitlin Macleod and Victoria McArthur argue, in their analysis of the respective interfaces of Tinder and Bumble, that 'gender is constructed within the apps both implicitly and explicitly' (2018, 823). They note that while gender is 'intrinsic to the technical aspects of the apps, Bumble and Tinder structure it in a way that is useful to their design rather than accommodating of nuanced and varied lived experiences of gender' (2018, 836): a flattening function with normative implications (see also David & Cambre, 2016). Stefanie Duguay notes that, because Tinder relies on Facebook as a kind of guarantor that users on the app are authentic, it benefits from Facebook fostering presentable users who abide by norms, and it draws a direct line between authenticity and normativity in its marketing materials by emphasising young white heterosexual people. Kenneth Hanson (2021) has also found that app use among heterosexual college students reinforces whiteness and gendered norms. Even on apps that target LGBTQ+ users, such as Grindr, an app predominantly for gay men, heteronormativity is evident, with users often rejecting potential partners who do not fit a normative ideal, in that they might be 'older, black, short, fat, with long hair, and, mainly, …effeminate' (Saraiva et al., 2020, 127). Similarly, a study of bisexual women using Tinder in New Zealand found that these users were positioned 'as "outsiders" in a heteronormative and biphobic domain' (Pond & Farvid, 2017, 20).

The gendered scripts and attitudes expressed in, via and around dating apps are necessarily inflected with place. This is another foundational aspect to dating app algorithms – they are location-aware, as they seek to match users with prospective partners in the same geographical radius. There can be distinct differences in the ways people use dating apps at home versus when they are travelling: for instance, when travelling in an unfamiliar city, users might feel a lot more free in their app use than in a small town where they live, where they run a much higher risk of encountering people they know on the app. As Condie, Lean and James argue, 'location and place are central to how you use Tinder [and, we contend, other dating apps as well] and who you can be there' (2018, 109). This becomes particularly important during a period like the 2020 pandemic lockdowns, where travel was virtually impossible. For the most part, people were engaging with apps in their 'home' rather than 'travel' mode, but there was an added layer of difficulty, as even though they might meet people on the app who lived in close proximity, opportunities to physically meet were extremely limited.

The notion of sexual scripting was developed by sociologists John H. Gagnon and William Simon in the 1970s and has been refined over the ensuing decades (1973, 1986, 1987, 1990, 2003). These scripts are 'socially learned narratives that govern the way people approach their sex lives, in addition to or instead of biological imperatives' (McAlister, 2020, 10). This is deeply bound up with gender – as Gagnon and Simon note, 'the sexual also shares the burden of demonstrating social, gender, and moral competence' (1986, 116) – and thus sexual scripts 'help to dictate and shape "appropriate" masculine and feminine roles that men and women may play in heterosexual romantic relationships' (Albright & Carter, 2019, 13; see also Comunello et al., 2020). Within these scripts, there must be room for agency, improvisation, critique, digression, rejection, appropriation and beyond, as articulated within this research.

In collecting this research, several gendered and culturally specific notions emerged, including ideas of the 'Aussie Bloke' and of the 'High-Maintenance Girl'. In examining these ideas, and understanding the limitations, subversions, and continuities that occurred, I referred to Linzi Murrie's work on the Aussie Bloke, and the Australian identity as being linked to masculinity, as well as McRobbie's investigation of the 'Alpha girl' and other genders romantic master tropes. I was interested in the way users mobilised or dispelled know relationship milestones and narrative theory in scripting their own love narratives in the online environment. The presence of a clear romance masterplot in the way users navigated their dating app experience was undeniable. According to Peter Brooks (1996, p. 19):

> Our very definition as human beings is very much bound up with the stories we tell about our own lives and the world in which we live. We cannot, in our dreams, our daydreams, our ambitious fantasies, avoid the imaginative imposition of form on life. Life is in many respects narrativized in series and bunches of intersecting stories – never complete until our death, of course, but nonetheless oriented toward the significant chaptalization of our existence. The presence of this chaptalization, and romantic story-telling in dating app user practices was clear, and will later be explored. Whether this story-telling was exacerbated by the uncertainty of Covid-19 is questionable, as there is no other comparative data.

Springboarding from Zygmunt Bauman's (2003) concept of 'Liquid Love', the notion that modernity produces are specific romantic condition, where lovers are tying bonds loosely with the express intent of unloosening them once a more formidable match presents itself (Bauman indicates computer dating as a specific example of this condition), Dr. Jodi McAlister and I developed an idea – Jagged Love (2021) – that focused on the anxiety, stress and even extreme emotions users experienced when using dating apps during COVID-19. Jagged

Love manifested cyclically, as participants turned to the apps seeking the security offered by the romance masterplots in a time of global uncertainty; swiped, matched, and messaged in large numbers, and lost faith in the apps ability to deliver on the romantic masterplots. While episodic behaviour on dating apps is not new, the pandemic heightened and accelerated the process as people desperately sought the certainty offered by the romance masterplots, quickly lost faith because of the limitations of the pandemic, and then returned again.

The extreme emotions experienced by users in their dating app use seemed to counteract any ideas that a durable intimacy cannot be developed in the digital domain. Indeed questions around IRL intimacy and digital intimacies have long been debated by scholars – often with the flavour that intimacies developed in the digital domain aren't as 'wholesome' as those developed in the physical space. For Berlant (1998), intimacy is created through the sharing of details inward to the self, or indeed creating a shared trajectory into the future with the other person. It quickly became clear in this research that users simply did not share enough to create intimacy, that their intermittent use of dating apps and their protective strategies of 'keeping their numbers high' often resulted in shallow and low-level intimacies, but not less hurt. The behaviours ran counter-productive to their romantic desires.

Here, I seek to respond to the need for more in-depth analysis of dating app use and its impact on intimacy and heteronormativity. Often dating apps are positioned in a highly polarised space – they are viewed as noxious for intimacy or romance, modern-day love villains, or worse, amplifiers of sexual assault and archaic gender scripts. My aim was to examine the nuances that existed within the dating app and intimacy space, by seeking out how dating apps continued and subverted gendered relationship stereotypes, by testing the limits and possibilities of agency within the digital landscape, the enacted romantic mastertropes and shifts, the disjunctures and continuities. By merging together dating app and intimacy scholarship, as well as the existing media and social dialogue, I sought to gather a more graduated and varied analysis of the impact of dating apps on intimacy. In particular, I look to disturb the idea that a single master trope is produced, or way of doing gender, or manner in which participants used or were restricted by dating apps – and instead, I seek to reinforce the open-mindedness, the multiplicity, the process and the intricateness of romantic mastertropes, dating apps, and gender scripts. At the same time drawing out the impact of COVID-19 in this process of love and intimacy making. I hope you enjoy the chapters to come. The ideas contained are intended to be complex, even at times contradictory. When you deal with human beings, you deal with a constant state of becoming, a multiplicity of at times inconsistent, and often clashing truths, which sit side-by-side often in inharmonious ways. It was my job to do justice to these ideas – rather than explain them in neat and rational ways. So yes, the ideas contained here are messy, but so are we all, especially when we deal with the ambit of love.

2

SOCIAL CONTEXT

We don't come to our dating app use, or even, our negotiations of love, as though from a void. We have pre-existing ideas on the topics which act as a fulcrum for how we interact with the apps, and indeed other people. Whilst conducting this research, a media dialogue swirled around the safety of dating apps, and at the same time, the media reported about their fervent usage. This chapter contextualises the pre-existing knowledge users had as they entered the dating app and intimacy domain in 2020. In particular, I use one case study, a Four Corners story that garnered widespread media attention in 2020 to describe the flavour of media reporting at the time. There were several large holes in the reporting, which seemed to invite the condemnation of dating apps, as the source of growing sexual assault numbers in Australia. In particular, the story focused on the safety (or lack thereof) of women on dating apps – quietly, and ever so stealthy, removing sexual agency from many women. Much dating app reporting tends to contain misinformation, and it's unclear whether or not this is because the reporting is intentionally sensationalised as click-bait, or indeed if the journalists involved have never used dating apps (and hence report distortions). *Indeed, dating apps form part of a cloistered world.* Unlike Facebook or Instagram, you simply can't google dating apps and have an insiders look – without an account, you'll never fully experience the dating app maelstrom.

Second, I'll describe the other media messaging tranche which proliferated during COVID-19, which focused on the massive jump in dating app usage worldwide. The media (including myself) reported against immense surges in downloads, but also usage including swiping and direct messages. Whilst we hypothesised the rationale for this usage, it was difficult to isolate the cause: was it a fear of loneliness (for those told to socially isolate alone)? Was it the COVID time compression accordion – which appeared to make people feel

DOI: 10.4324/9781003120353-2

stuck in inertia, desperate to reach life milestones or a sense that they were moving forward? Was it pragmatic? That is, dating apps were the only way users in lockdown could meet during COVID-19. Or finally, was it FOMO? The fear of missing out – driven by an incessant media dialogue, which indicated everyone was on dating apps? All of which will be explored in later changes. At this stage, I'll simply provide an indication of the media reporting.

Finally, in the last section, I'll also describe dating app functionality and background, using Tinder and Bumble as case studies, to allow the reader further context on the dating apps.

Case study 1 – patriarchal reporting

In October 2020, Four Corners aired a programme that investigated Tinder titled: 'Tinder and how digital dating became a predators' playground' (ABC, 2020). The investigation was a collaboration with Triple J Hack and purported to 'reveal that the dating app was a playground for sexual offenders' (ABC, 2020). In advance of the report, Four Corners and Triple J Hack put a call out to find people who had 'safety concerns' around dating apps. In total, 400 people responded. Out of these 231 people had used Tinder and of these, 48 people indicated they had experienced sexual violence from a person they had met on Tinder – this might include abusive messages, images or physical violence (ABC, 2020).

The programme, which aired on October 10, 2020, created widespread community condemnation of Tinder (ABC, 2020). News outlets like news.com (2020) and Mamamia (2020) followed suit with stories around the 'dark side of Tinder'. Junkee ran a story with the headline, 'Absolutely Sickening' (Junkee, 2020). Buried deep within the report was the core element – that 48 people had reported sexually abusive behaviours on Tinder, but only 11 of those people had received a response (ABC, 2020). The kernel of the story related to the way Tinder dealt with sexual abuse reports, and the organisation's willingness to collaborate with authorities within the justice space.

However, this story was enveloped by a broader narrative: Tinder is not a safe place for women.

The article and programme featured all female case studies – in particular, two women who were raped by men they had met on Tinder (ABC, 2020). The faces of women who had provided their testimonics were used to illustrate the article (some blurred out). The associated ABC digital news article drew out the specifics relating to one case (ABC, 2020). The woman described she had matched with the rapist on Tinder and had agreed to meet with him, not knowing his surname, mobile number or any other personal details. The media release issues by Four Corners/Triple J Hack led with a quote from a father:

> It's like a minefield … It's a perfect platform for predators and scammers.
>
> *(ABC, 2020)*

It was unclear whether this 'father' had used Tinder, or where this information was gleaned from. However, Four Corners/Triple J Hack positioned this quote as the lead statement, above the testimony of women who had been raped.

In surfacing this story – Four Corners and Triple J Hack sought to expose the predatory nature of Tinder and, to some extent, empower women by telling their stories. But, there was nothing empowering in the story-telling. Recounting a story where a woman had been raped after she had met a man on Tinder, and not secured any of his personal details, *invited the flagrant questioning of her character.* Positioning a father's voice as the key statement, indicated to the reader that a man's voice (even one that had never used the dating app before) was the most important and legitimate source. The act of not describing how dating logistics are navigated in the online domain seemed an attempt to only narrate parts of the story, and those which built an argument in relation to women being unsafe on Tinder. Alongside this, the absence of statistics that would have described the nature of sexual assault in Australia (a broader discussion – not simply reducible to just Tinder) appeared as another aberration. Similarly, the singular focus on women, without attention on other vulnerable groups (like non-binary members of the community) or reference to points of intersectionality (for example, Indigenous, Culturally and Linguistically Diverse, queer or even remote or regional Australians), another omission. This package highlighted how contemporary media focus conflates intimacy and sex with danger and violence specifically within the dating app space.

In 2021, Australia experienced its own #metoo movement, after Brittany Higgins, former Liberal Party staffer, came forward, describing how she had been raped by the acting chief of staff of the then Defence Minister's Office, Linda Reynolds, in Parliament House in the lead up to the 2018 election (The Conversation, 2021). Higgins, at the time, reported the rape, only to be silenced by critical figures within the political system (The Conversation, 2021). Following Higgins' testimony, a series of other women came forward with similar reports (BBC, 2021). The Australian political system was rocked and a light shone on the violent misogyny which was occurring at the highest echelons. Women across Australia came forward with their stories, which culminated in the Justice Marches which happened across Australian capital cities (BBC, 2021). In light of these occurrences, and this reckoning, it's hard to imagine the Four Corners and Triple J Hack story running in 2021 – as it has now become abundantly clear that Tinder is not the genesis or only perpetrating force of sexual assault in Australia – and that indeed, sexual assault occurs within places where we would expect the highest levels of integrity (like federal Parliament House). In addition, it is not limited to interactions with strangers (as implied in the Four Corners and Triple J Hack – via the woman who had not collected the details of her rapist in advance of meeting him).

The story indicated that message threads could be deleted on Tinder, making it difficult to surface evidence relating to rape or sexual abuse (ABC, 2020). This is a common feature on many messaging and social media platforms, including, for example, Instagram, WhatsApp and iPhone messaging. The news programme did not indicate that most people progress the 'date logistics' on a separate platform to Tinder, for example, WhatsApp or Instagram (which, as indicated, have similar deletion features), or that in relation to the sending and receipt of explicit images, Tinder has no image send functionality (hence explicit images are sent or received on other platforms). Instead, the programme and associated articles positioned Tinder as the genesis or exacerbator of sexual abuse – or as titled, a 'predator's playground' (ABC, 2020).

Why was Tinder in particular, within a suite of other dating apps, situated at the priority focus for this story? In addition, why was Tinder positioned as the genesis of sexual assault or a 'predators playground'? And why were women situated as vulnerable (incapable of gathering vital details to ensure their own sexual protection) within the reporting? Finally, why was the legitimate source a 'Father'?

Applying Briggs and Hallin's theory of biocommunicability (2010) – which proposes that contemporary health professionals' scientific framing of public health problems is, in part, shaped by popular media discourses – Albury et al. (2020) identify the cross-over between dating app reporting and public health policy, noting that the dating app hysteria, often deployed by contemporary media leeks into public health policy, and more broadly general public understanding of dating apps. Albury et al. (2020) further note that this reporting of dating apps is often conducted by journalists who have never engaged with dating apps – unlike social media platforms such as Facebook or Instagram, dating apps aren't open for general public perusal. To navigate a dating app, like Bumble and Tinder, the user/or reporter must actively sign up, download, establish a profile and engage in online dating. As will later be identified, dating app use and the intimacy experienced are uniquely singular. Unlike other social networks, visibility is limited. As identified by Albury, Pym and McCosker, this lack of dating app understanding contributes to the widespread media hysteria in relation to usage. However, they identify a significant category of supportive discussions of safer app use within social news and lifestyle reporting. This discursive space features what they term as 'vernacular pedagogies' of app use, revealing app users' safety strategies and their experiences of pleasure and playfulness. They argue that an analysis of popular media can provide valuable insights into how everyday experiences of safety, risk and wellbeing are being shaped and contested with dating and hookup app use and that these insights can be used to develop meaningful health promotion strategies.

The Four Corners example story serves to highlight a couple of issues in dating app reporting. It tends to position dating apps (and in this case Tinder) as the genesis of sexual assault in Australia, again, proving the perpetrators with an easy no-responsibility escape route. Dating apps don't facilitate sexual assault, perpetrators do. In addition, the reporting is flagrantly patriarchal and indicates that women are 'at risk' on dating apps (evidenced through the father quote). Clearly, putting women's sexual agency into question. In addition, for the most part, it featured white women, ignoring ideas expressed by academics such as Carlson (2020), which indicate that the people most at risk on dating apps are vulnerable communities, Indigenous people, people of colour, ethnically diverse groups and LGBTIQ+ people. And, whilst I don't seek to fetishise dating apps, a more nuanced examination of the platforms, and how people use them is required.

As previously indicated, to delve further into this topic, you need an understanding of the apps themselves and their functionalities. Whilst there is a plethora of dating apps currently available to users, I chose to focus my work on Bumble and Tinder, for reasons I will expand on shortly.

Case study 2 – COVID

This research was collected during the first half of 2020 – which coincided with the start of the COVID-19 pandemic and lockdown in NSW. This meant that participants were in a unique dating paradigm – the digital domain represented the only space in which singles could mingle. Of course, this wasn't just dating apps – participants within my research indicated they were sliding into people's DMs via Instagram, SnapChat, TikTok or even LinkedIn.

However, in March 2020 (the start of lockdown in NSW) the hyper-usage of dating apps became a key media tranche of conversation.

The discussion commenced in the media and subsequently exploded across popular culture, on March 3, 2020, when Tinder issued an in-app public service announcement (PSA) regarding COVID-19. This was greeted with a panoply of memes and gags across social and mainstream media (The Project, March 5, 2020).

The Tinder PSA read:

> "Your Being Is Our #1 Priority"
>
> "Tinder is a great place to meet new people. While we want you to continue to have fun, protecting yourself from the Coronavirus is more important. Here are some of the tips to keep in mind:
>
> - Wash your hands frequently
> - Carry hand sanitizer
> - Avoid touching your face
> - Maintain social distance in public gatherings."

Tinder then provided its users with a link directing them to the World Health Organization (WHO) website. Bumble's company spokespeople spoke directly with TMZ, revealing that their global customer service team has directing their users to the CDC and WHO sites for up-to-date info on the current coronavirus pandemic.

Suddenly, dating apps were front and centre in the media, and within the social media barrage. Twitter became a haven for comments such as, 'When Tinder turns into your household doctor, you know you're in trouble'.

This intense media focus, coincided with an uplift in app usage number – as described by Dietzel, Myers and Duguay (2021) in The Conversation as a significant shift in usage and behaviour:

> This shift has increased the number of dating app users and the amount of time people spend on dating apps. Tinder says its users had 11 per cent more swipes and 42 per cent more matches last year, making 2020 the apps busiest app.

Between March 5 and 10, OkCupid reported a 7 percent increase in new conversations, and at the same time, 10 out of the top 100 apps on the iTunes Store were dating apps (Portolan, The Conversation, 2020). During the second week of March, active users on Bumble rose by 8 percent. As American cities went into lockdown, apps reported increased numbers of messaging. On Bumble from March 12 to 22, Seattle saw a 23 percent increase in sent messages, New York City 23 percent and San Francisco 26 percent. This was a trend that was reported worldwide – with the then CEO of Tinder, Elie Seidman (The Verve, 2020), indicating the rise of an episodic use of dating apps, which coincided with cities going into lockdown. Dating apps, however, are intended to facilitate a face-to-face meeting, which was no longer possible within the COVID-19 lockdown landscape. Dating apps sought to facilitate this shift in interactions, by catering to a largely digital paradigm. For example, Tinder and Bumble introduced video chat capabilities.

Social media also pointed to another interesting trend: DM chats were becoming largely COVID-centric. In the month of March OkCupid reported a 188 percent increase in the number of profiles that mentioned COVID-19. Indian Tinder users also described a rise in longer DM chats, and media started to report this as a return to a Jane-Austen-like style of courtships. COVID-19 threatened to flatten the casual hook-up, and instead re-instate the old-school romance of a Jane-Austen-Esque world. Instead of love letters, video and DM chats were the new forms of dialogue within these dating app courtships.

Indeed, I weighed into the media debate, with my own articles in The Conversation, The New Daily and even spots on daytime television. Here's what I had to say:

> In this new world, we're all navigating how romantic intimacy can exist without physical contact.
>
> With the prospect of months of self-isolation how will we navigate sex? After all, not everyone has a sexual partner readily available.
>
> A notice about sex and coronavirus from the New York City Department of Health went viral last weekend. It included the statement "You are your safest sex partner".
>
> The tables are suddenly turned: online hook-ups were previously framed as less wholesome than face-to-face ones. Yet in 2020 they are perceived as safer.

> Connection is sought after in times of uncertainty, risk and crisis. But COVID-19 makes the navigation of these intimacies certainly difficult. We are in the middle of a historical re-jigging of our understanding of romance, intimacy and sex.
>
> It's safe to say the negotiation of intimacy has been irrevocably changed – even if it is only for the short while.

It was an incredibly topical issue – however, unknowingly, did we drive this usage fervour in reporting about the surge in numbers and hypothesising as to why? And did we similarly drive a sense of FOMO, a need to participate or drop out of the love-making scene for the COVID-lockdown period (timeframe unknown)?

I will explore this later – however, it's safe to say there were two key tranches of media framing user experience during COVID lockdown:

1. Patriarchal reporting (moral panic about dating apps and their impact on love, romance and dating, as well as safety implications);
2. Immense surges in usage (FOMO, get in there or lose out).

Importantly, this is the lens through which participants (users) approached my research.

Next, onto the dating apps themselves.

The dating apps: Bumble and Tinder

Speaking broadly, a dating app is an app whose purpose is to facilitate its user to find a partner. The word 'partner' is used loosely here, as this could span anything from a short-term connection or hook-up to a long-term romantic relationship. Not all apps are designed for the same purpose, not all users use them in the same way and not all users use them in the way the app is designed. Some users use apps designed to find hookups to find long-term partners, some do the inverse and some maintain different profiles on a given app seeking different things (e.g. a 'hook-up profile' and a 'relationship profile').

Whilst many dating apps exist and are accessible to the Australian market, the rationale for selecting Bumble and Tinder as the case studies for my research related to how they seemingly form the male and female sides of the (extraordinarily binary) dating app coin. Seemingly, the two apps represent the character traits associated with 'toxic masculinity' (Tinder) and hyper-femininity (Bumble). According to participants and the media, Tinder is 'hard and fast', a 'meat market' and even a 'predators' playground' – whilst Lee (2019) identified Bumble as speaking to a 'polite courtship' where men are identified as a potential threat and as a result policed from making the first (and implicitly predatory) move. Indeed, this is an incredibly surface read of the apps – and as we'll discover, often incorrect, however, this imagined duality fueled the selection.

Bumble is careful to state that the relationships it seeks to facilitate are more than simply romantic: nominally, the app 'allows you to feel empowered while you make those connections, whether you're dating, looking for friends, or growing your professional network', and sells itself as 'where people go to learn how to establish and maintain healthier connections' (Bumble n.d.). Tinder is more explicit that its purpose is 'bringing singles together online', but notes that this does not necessarily have to be for long-term relationships: it notes that while other apps are designed specifically for this purpose, they are 'all about the experience and offer possibilities for whatever it is you're looking for'. Many participants in my study maintained profiles on both apps, as well as one or more other apps, some reading with the grain of the app's expressed purpose, some against it and some somewhere between the two poles. In short, this is complex terrain, and apps are complicated assemblages that can be many things to many people. As Jenna Condie, Garth Lean and Donna James write of Tinder, any given dating app can be 'a way-finder, knowledge-generator, friendship-giver, sex-sorter, game-changer, time-passer, soul-destroyer, esteem-giver, self-depressor, sushi-train, love-machine' (2018, 112).

Both apps can also be seen as targeted towards the heterosexual masses (Bertoni, 2014; Duguay). As Duguay identifies, Tinder, '... directly targets heterosexual users and has garnered the participation of large number of heterosexual users'. Tinder was the first location-based mobile dating app to receive rapid uptake in the heterosexual market, reaching more than 15 million matches per day in 2014 just two years after its launch (Bertoni, 2014), and today reaches approximately 65 million worldwide. It is a common tool for navigating intimate life in Australia (Newett et al., 2017). It is the ubiquity of Tinder, as well as its prominence within the heterosexual market, and its reputational 'bro' factor which made it a pertinent 'case study' for this research (Jin, 2019).

However, contemporary media has worked hard to establish Tinder as the bro app and Bumble, the feminist app. Tinder has sought to distance the brand from a 'bro' and hook-up reputation, seeking to position itself with a space of 'connection'. In contrast, Bumble has courted its feminist vibe with CEO Whitney Wolfe Herd saying that Bumble is '100 percent a feminist app' in an interview with Vanity Fair in 2015. This 'feminist app' status has been challenged across the last six years, both from an academic and contemporary media perspective – with journalists labelling it a 'gimmick' and academics such as Bivens and Hoque (2018) challenging the type of feminism it champions (white, cis-gender). Bumble itself in recent years has stepped away from the overt use of the word 'feminist'. The word no longer appears in marketing collateral (such as its website or social platforms), instead, the following tagline is deployed to describe the Bumble business – 'There is no equality without respect, and that's where all healthy relationships start. To challenge outdated heterosexual norms, women make the first move on Bumble (Bumble, official website, 2021)'. With over 3.5 million registered users, Bumble's marketing, content and messaging are often unabashedly heterosexual, despite its proclaimed values of sexual diversity and inclusivity Bivens and Hoque (2018).

Bumble and Tinder are two of the largest and most prevalent dating apps in the market at the time, and they have an implicit relationship, in that their designers and owners were linked. As previously indicated, Tinder was the first heterosexual dating app to hit the market in 2011 and achieve levels of market ubiquity. Co-founder Whitney Wolfe Herd went on to create Bumble alongside Andrey Andreev (CEO of Badoo) following a Tinder sexual harassment claim. Reportedly, the suit was settled outside of court to the tune of 1 million USD (Forbes, 2018). The two dating apps have continued their hostile relationship since, with Tinder counter-suing Bumble around the use of their signature swipe functionality. However, when Bumble was publicly floated in 2021, Tinder or Tinder owner match.com sought to acquire the app as part of their broader dating app stable which includes Hinge.

Tinder: the background

Tinder is considered to be the most popular dating app for iOS and Android with at least 10 million users a day (Ayers, 2014; Freier, 2015). The most powerful tool within Tinder's marketing arsenal is its ubiquity. On its website Tinder proclaims that it reaches some 194 countries around the world – which is significant given that there are 195 recognised countries in the world today (this comprises of 193 countries that are member states of the United Nations and 2 countries that are non-member observer states: the Holy See and the State of Palestine. It is reasonable to assume that the Holy See is the member state which Tinder currently does not operate within). This makes the app virtually omnipresent, and as a result users often download Tinder because of its market majority.

Tinder was created by Hatch Labs, the start-up incubator run by InterActiveCorp (the parent company of Match Group), Hatch Labs. Sean Rad (former CEO and chairman) and Justin Mateen (former CMO) are seen as the key collaborators in developing Tinder. Notably, InterActiveCorp (IAC) is also responsible for other dating apps besides Match.com and Tinder, including OkCupid and Zhenai (China), demonstrating the centralising economic and socialising force of a large corporate. Tinder, like Facebook, was initially trialed in a series of US college campuses, and then rolled out to almost instant expansion, achieving 350 million swipes per day by late 2013, and rising to one billion swipes per day before the end of 2014. The premium subscription model (later to be described) was added in 2015, and Tinder Gold was included in 2017.

Tinder currently boasts 57 million users around the world, and 5.9 million Tinder subscribers pay for premium Tinder Plus and Tinder Gold. Recent Tinder statistics indicate that Tinder users, on average, log in four times a day, and are most active after 9 pm. Tinder's estimated market worth is $10 billion as of March 2020, parent group, Match is worth $18.6 million.

Tinder continues to grow Year-On-Year (YOY), in terms of usage rates, and similarly, its paid subscriber usage rate continues to grow.

Tinder does not reveal its demographic breakdown, except to indicate that half of its users belong to Generation Z – that is those born from the early to mid-90s. Available Tinder statistics for Australia date back to 2015, however, a snapshot from Statista offers a view of Tinder's nationality user break-down in terms of revenue, with Australia positioned as four behind the US, the UK and Canada. Noting that the four top countries are English-speaking 'western' nations, however, this data reflects revenue based on premium packages and could reflect multiple trends, such as nations more willing to pay for relationship/hook-up success, etc.

In summary, Tinder's ubiquity is revealed through these statistics, but also the homogenising force and data power of InterActiveCorp in the dating market (parent company: Tinder, match.com and OkCupid). Alongside this, the intensity of individual usage is highlighted (through average number of per day log-ins, matches and swipes per year).

Bumble (the background)

The dating app Bumble was founded in December 2014 by Whitney Wolfe Herd (a co-creator of Tinder), in Austin, Texas. The app is a female focussed dating app and provides women with the power to make the first move, or start the DM discussion, reframing powerful narratives around men taking the lead in relationships.

The company is closely linked to Wolfe Herd and her own assent in the tech landscape – a largely 'brogrammer' and misogynistic space. At 22, Wolfe Herd joined Hatch Labs and was involved with the start-up Cardify, a project led by Sean Rad through Hatch Labs IAC incubator. This project was later abandoned and she joined the Tinder development team with Rad and Chris Gulczynski in 2012. Wolfe Herd became the Vice President of Tinder marketing and has been largely credited for the Tinder logo (which is based on kindling and a flame) and also for its success on college campuses. However, Wolf Herd left the company in 2014 after growing tensions with executives, and later filed a sexual harassment suit against Tinder and Sean Rad, and reportedly received more than $1 million in Tinder stocks as part of the settlement.

Bumble was created alongside Andrey Andreev, founder of Badoo, and is part of the stable of dating apps owned by parent company MagicLab, which was sold to the private equity firm the BlackStone Group in November 2019. Co-founder Andreev relinquished his entire stake in both Bumble and Badoo and Wolfe Herd was made the CEO of the newly acquired MagicLab, then valued at $3 million with an estimated 75 million users. Badoo was later the subject of a Forbes investigation reporting workplace misogyny, drug use, sexual assault and racial discrimination.

The mandate established from the onset for Bumble was a 'female focussed' dating app, which provided women with the power to navigate and negotiate relationships on their own terms.[1] This came with the advantage of 'weeding out creeps', and avoiding the 'harassment' that women might experience on other dating apps (for example the sending of unsolicited sexually explicit images, or constant and explicit messaging).[2] Bumble and Wolfe Herd have recently spearheaded legislation which makes the sending of unsolicited explicit imagery illegal in the US. In March 2019, Wolfe Herd testified before the Texas House Criminal Jurisprudence committee about the prevalence of unsolicited explicit photos sent to female users on dating applications, and later legislation was passed in Texas which makes the sending of unsolicited explicit images illegal.[3] Wolfe Herd also has a stake in the US-based dating app, Chappy, which was co-founded by Jack Rogers, Max Cheremkin and Ollie Locke.[4]

The key points of difference for Bumble include:

- Women on the app are required to make the first move;
- There is a 24-hour clock that starts ticking from the moment two people match, the discussion must commence within these 24 hours otherwise the match is removed; and
- The dating app funnels the user into finding a BFF, a business or a relationship from the onset via a widget functionality.

There are other secondary points of difference in the premium model, which will be articulated in the Tinder comparative table.

In November 2019, Bumble reported 3 million Australian users, and at the time boasted 70 million users world-wide. Michelle Battersby, Bumble publicist at the time indicated:

> 'It attracts women who want to make that first move and men who respect that in women. It means from the moment you're matching with someone, there's a different tone for the conversation.' (Sydney Morning Herald, November, 2019.) She went onto say: 'It's great to instil that kind of behaviour in women's minds. You shouldn't have to wait for opportunities to come to you – if it's in dating, don't be afraid to speak to a guy; if it's for an opportunity, don't be afraid to pursue it.'

Bumble's ethos of independent women, and women that get things done is very reminiscent of a 'lean in' argument which was popular in silicon valley and was particularly embodied via then COO Sheryl Sandberg. Launched during the height of the #metoo movement and certainly received much critical media success and was described as a 'women's movement' and 'empowering'.

Bumble and Tinder: key functionality similarities and differences

Overall, Bumble and Tinder are incredibly similar. They function off the basis of a swipe right/left basis and are image-led. Whilst Bumble allows for a greater description and badges to show in a snapshot whether you're an atheist, smoker, Vegan or even, if you're COVID vaccinated. Both have a base service, which can be upgraded to a Plus or Gold service. For example, Tinder Plus and Tinder Gold provide the user the ability to **like** a profile, this means the user knows who has already liked their profile before making a decision on swiping right or left. The **Tinder Rewind** feature allows you to undo a mistake i.e. it lets you take back your last Like of Nope. If you accidentally passed on someone you wanted to get to know. **Tinder Passport** allows you to like, match and chat with others around the world by simply searching for a city or dropping a pin on the map. Notably, Tinder provided everyone with a free passport during COVID to find quarantine buddies. You can also **Boost** your account on Tinder which will be of the top profiles in the area for 30 mins. Bumble has a 24-hour clock, which creates some impetus for action. That means if you've matched with someone, there are 24 hours in which a woman can start the conversation before the match disappears. Bumble also offers other serves such as Bumble Business or Bumble BFF, for those looking for friends or Business connections. Obviously, the key point of difference is that women have to start the chat on Bumble as opposed to Tinder, where either party can start the conversation.

The reality is, if you've never used a dating apps, you can never fully understand the experience. This is part of the dating app strategy – either participate or no cigar. It is a cloistered world – even to users (as we'll later discover – who never really get to compare the experience, and for the most part, have to rely on their own radar to gather an understanding of what they're doing wrong, or right.

Notes

1 Bumble.com
2 Bumble.com
3 https://www.dallasnews.com/business/technology/2019/03/26/bumble-founder-wants-texas-lawmakers-to-make-unwanted-sexting-a-crime/
4 https://www.statesman.com/business/20191111/blackstone-to-buy-owner-of-austinrsquos-bumble-and-chappy-dating-apps

3

JAGGED LOVE – THE CONFLICT

Romance vs dating apps

The dating app domain has often been framed as a location for hook-ups – for quick, transactional, no-strings-attached sex (Bryden, 2017). Whilst some researchers have challenged this idea, describing a fluidity of desires and practices on dating apps (Albury, 2020), the hook-up dating app narrative has remained prevalent in contemporary culture. Researchers such as Bauman have described the world of computer-mediated dating as synonymous with 'Liquid Love' – a type of a fleeting love, where bonds are tied loosely, prepared from the onset for dissolution. Bauman contends that the dating app scene presents a rotating door of potential partners – where one is always looking for the someone better who might appear at the next swipe. However, the majority of participants within this research sample were seeking monogamous, long-term relationships via dating apps, and even those, who sought hook-ups, framed their discussions in terms of 'keeping their eyes on the prize' (which was, the monogamous relationship). In this chapter, I examine how participants often mobilised relationship narratives in describing their dating app usage, and what they were looking for in a relationship, and if this was impacted by the COVID-19 lockdown. For example, participants often described the narrative 'meet-cute', or the concept of 'the one', and leant heavily on references to Hollywood rom-coms, to provide background to their romanticism.

There was an order and process required for the progression of romantic relationships, which often conflicted with the information architecture of dating apps. Tinder and Bumble were described as 'sterile' and 'mechanical' spaces which didn't encourage the kind of romantic narrative participants sought. This is not to say that there is only *one* romantic narrative, or that this version of the narrative wasn't challenged by participants (for example, the consensually non-monogamous couple who participated in the research). Nor does it purport that all participants were looking for a romantic companion on dating apps.

DOI: 10.4324/9781003120353-3

However, there was a consistent pattern among the majority of participants in their desire to find a version of 'the one' and their own personal relationship matertrope(s) via dating apps – this search could have been exacerbated or cemented by the COVID-19 pandemic, the sense of uncertainty, as well as the dissolution of life milestones that the pandemic seemed to produce. It was impossible to ignore the impact of COVID-19 on the research outcomes, and it coloured the majority of dialogues.

I examine how Bauman's theory of Liquid Love, was bent, extended by participants and/or replaced by what I came to term 'Jagged Love' (alongside Dr Jodi McAlister) – a peculiar state, where participants described a certain dating online busy-ness, a desire for romantic/monogamous outcomes, strategic participation on dating apps and anxiety. The metaphor of liquid is an important one for Bauman. Relationships for him are like Cordial – currently taken undiluted, and while the hit is intoxicating, it is at the same time, nauseating. Bauman espouses that our deepest wish is to prevent our relationships from curdling and clotting, or becoming solid (that, we fear, is what marriages used to be about). Bauman imagines a world of SDCs (semi-detached couples), self-styled romantic revolutionaries who want separate pads from their partners and a Rolodex filled with ready lovers – liquid moderns. However, within this loose romantic paradigm we find ourselves anxious. Torn, as Freud recognised, between freedom and security. According to Bauman, those who tilt the balance too far to freedom, are often found rushing back home, desperate to be loved, eager to re-establish communities. But that's not to say that the liquid moderns want their old suffocating security back. They want the impossible: to have their cake and eat it, to be free and secure. And to some degree this paradigm was described by participants, this conflict between freedom and security, and yet, there was a deep yearning for security, and relationship security. Participants weren't liquid moderns, they were *solid-anxious-moderns*. They sought to trigger this sense of relationship security by setting a romantic narrative into motion – knocking one milestone down at a time, seemingly domino style. Only the dating app space didn't provide the necessary ingredients for this to occur.

In this chapter, I examine romantic narratives and how they were integrated, revolutionised, reshaped, restyled, chewed and regurgitated in different ways. As well as the conflict between Jagged and Liquid Love and the impact of the pandemic in driving a vociferous, condensed romantic narrative.

The pandemic – how COVID-19 condensed love, accordion style

Numerous studies, have been developed to identify how confinement has impacted the health of the world population, aiming at identifying possible relationships between psychosocial, psychological and behavioural changes during the confinement period and obtaining scientific data that could help to characterise the psychosocial aspects of the COVID-19 crisis (Ammar et al., 2020). In general, authors describe how the COVID-19 pandemic has impacted the mental health of citizens worldwide; isolation measures, fear, uncertainty, economic turmoil, lack of social connectedness and trust in other people and institutions, and jobs and incomes being at risk are taking a huge toll in terms of anxiety and worry, leading to 'psychological distress'. The United Nations (UN) has warned of the necessity for a policy briefing, calling for substantial investment in support services. Depression and anxiety cost the global economy more than one trillion dollars per year, and this was before the COVID-19 pandemic, and globally the ratio of mental health professionals per citizen is 1 to 10,000. It was impossible not to frame the research findings against and through the lens of the COVID-19 pandemic, as the data was collected during the first lockdown in NSW, and there was a clear interplay or correlation between the findings, and the pragmatic and psychosocial impacts of the pandemic.

Much discussion occurred in contemporary media around the connection between surges in dating app usage and COVID-19. As previously articulated, dating apps reported significant increases in new sign-ups, as well as swipes and DM chats during the pandemic. Elie Seidman, the CEO of Tinder (2020, The Verve) indicated, this growth tended to align with periods when cities went into lockdown, the spike was often followed by a trough, which coincided with the end of lockdown. This trend was observed across cities around the world, including Sydney (Seidman, The Verve, 2020). Logically, dating apps became one of the few locations where people could meet and connect. Other digital platforms like Instagram, and LinkedIn also became sites used for dating purposes, where the phenomena of 'sliding into' a romantic interests DMs was given a COVID twist (Portolan & McAlister, 2021). Pragmatically, COVID also drove a desire for many singles who lived alone to find an 'iso-partner'.

Participants described a sharp increase in matches and conversations at the beginning of the lockdown (March 2020). This included new users–as one participant said,

> This weird thing happened, where all of these new faces started popping up. Like before I was seeing repeats, the same people going around, but there was like … this influx of people.

Another indicated:

> My phone was pinging off the hook.

In reference to the alerts she was receiving from dating apps regarding matches, and DMs.

The start of the COVID-19 lockdown for singles living alone was particularly tough, as NSW government guidelines were based around the 'familial unit'. This meant that singles could only travel to see and connect with what was classed as a 'significant other'. The parameters around what constituted a 'significant other' were also loose and undefined – putting pressure on new relationships to establish a definition prematurely. During the second COVID-19 lockdown in Sydney (2021), the NSW Government introduced the concept of 'singles bubbles' – where singles could nominate one person to visit on an ongoing basis during the lockdown.

Undoubtably, lockdown had a significant impact on singles living alone across NSW. The majority of participants within the sample lived within shared homes, or with their parents. Three of the participants lived alone, two of which were single parents. These three participants were often more willing to try different technologies to connect, for example video-calls, or to experiment with dating styles aligned to NSW Government guidelines on COVID-socialising, like walking or park dates. One of these participants indicated:

> I really kind of liked the video chats. I did a few of them with different people … with one person I chatted to him for a couple of hours. We even did a Netflix and Uber eats thing where he ordered food to my door and we watched a movie and talked.

This was in contrast to participants who lived in a share home, or lived with parents, many of whom described video chats as creepy, or were unwilling to go on walking dates, and were more interested in 'waiting it out' to date post-pandemic. Single participants living alone often described the loneliness they experienced during lockdown, and it seemed they were hungrier to secure an iso-partner to share the lockdown period with.

> Sometimes I won't see anyone at all. It will just be me for days on end … I know you can talk to people on the phone, and zoom, but … it's actually really depressing.

Participants who lived with friends and family talked about the connection they experienced with these people during COVID, and how they had been instrumental to helping them get through. They also talked about how they were unwilling to go out and connect with a stranger they met online face-to-face for fear they might bring COVID back to loved ones.

> I live with my parents, and they're in their sixties … like I'm not that selfish. I'm not going to go out for the sake of a hook-up and then maybe bring Covid back into the home.

Hence, the desire to try new technologies via dating apps and connect face-to-face was driven largely from a pragmatic perspective. Alongside this pragmatism, participants expressed a sense of uncertainty, a scattering of life milestones and of purpose, which made them double-down on the idea of finding love or a romantic companion. One participant indicated:

> I've never cried so much before. I cry almost every day …. I just don't know what I'm doing, or what this means anymore.

Seemingly, the removal of daily routines, like work, the gym, even a morning coffee at the local cafe, scrambled participants sense of purpose and created a certain life inertia. A feeling that nothing was moving forward, that critical milestones weren't being met. Within this quagmire, participants sort to shift the traditional relationship milestone forward. A romantic companion was not only seen as something that would provide solace, but also as a milestone that could be reached during the pandemic, while the rest of their life was on hold. This sense of missed milestones, or level of introspection was keenly felt. One participant indicated:

> I definitely feel like I should have done more with my life by now. Like there's all these things that I *should* have sorted by now … the job, the house, the partner. It's like if one fell into place the others would … does that make sense?

This participant went onto say:

> Sometimes I think if I met that person, then my life would start … and then some times I think I don't need anyone at all. Like I'm an independent woman, I don't need a dude to like … you know …

For many participants there was a clear temporal anxiety embedded in their anxieties: a sense that they had begun falling behind, that the 'right time', as McLaren (1999) might put it, might be passing by. This seemed to be compounded by COVID-19, which appeared to compress time for participants accordion style. The Lockdown -Pandemic-Time conundrum in relation to the duration of time:

> One distinction is about the fact that judgments about the passage of time are not duration judgments (Droit-Volet and Wearden, 2015, 2016; Wearden, 2015). In the former case, one refers to judgments about how fast time seems to pass in some situations. What is referred to as duration judgments is the type of investigation based on an explicit judgment about the duration of an interval, or the duration of an activity or task. Both types of judgments are not related, according to Droit-Volet and Wearden (2016). The judgments about the passage of time are indeed closer to phenomenology and, as noted by Droit-Volet and Wearden (2016), these judgments are linked to the individuals' introspection on their internal life.

It was this introspection of their internal life, and the milestones which had been missed (particularly of the romantic companionate variety) which seemed to impact participants the most, and drive them towards seeking outcomes (or a relationship) via a dating app. However, the form and shape of this relationship were very much set and standardised and drew heavily on versions of the romantic masterplot(s). Not all participants followed suit, however, the sense of uncertainty seemed to impact their relationship statuses, or reflection on their relationship statuses in interesting ways – for example the consensually non-monogamous couple became monogamous during the pandemic, and those looking for hook-ups slowed their hook-up pace (or stopped hooking-up all together). The liquid modern was indeed brought under attack by the pandemic and replaced by a *desire* for solidity.

Relationship narratives invoked to stabilise the ship

In a time of global uncertainty, participants turned to the apps seeking the security offered by the romance masterplot(s). As previously described, the romantic masterplot(s) is one of the most obvious examples of a masterplot in contemporary Western culture is the romance plot. This is a plot into which many people inscribe themselves, and it has become one of the primary ways in which people narrativise their lives. Romance plots are visible in the vast majority of the media we consume and have become 'culturally sanctioned templates for interpreting reality around us' (Roche et al., 2018, 36). The plot has clear milestones and events: you meet someone, you fall in love, you marry, you have children and you live happily ever after. These milestones are flexible and might shift in terms of significance and order – for instance, not all couples marry, have children or wait until after marriage to have children – but the cultural primacy of the romance plot, and our almost universal familiarity with it, cannot be denied. This master plot has consistently been challenged, subverted, reinterpreted and even bent. However, it was persistently regurgitated by participants within this research sample, in different and interesting ways. In reference to romantic masterplot(s), the timing of specific relationship milestones is particularly relevant, as this was of particular relevance in relation to the time accordion and COVID-19. Other studies, relating to gender and the interpretation of masterplot(s), for example, Smith's work on consumer culture, gender and masterplot(s) is more relevant to the gendered ways users presented themselves in the dating app environment (Chapter 7). In relation to masterplot(s) and milestones, I particularly focus on concepts of 'straight-time' as defined in Chapter 1. Questions of gender and sexuality are fundamental to dating apps. It is foundational to app algorithms, as this is the key way in which a user indicates their preference as to whose profiles the app will show them. There have been several studies examining apps through the lens of gender. Caitlin Macleod and Victoria McArthur argue, in their analysis of the respective interfaces of Tinder and Bumble, that 'gender is constructed within the apps both implicitly and explicitly' (2018, 823).

They note that while gender is 'intrinsic to the technical aspects of the apps, Bumble and Tinder structure it in a way that is useful to their design rather than accommodating of nuanced and varied lived experiences of gender' (2018, 836): a flattening function with normative implications (see also David & Cambre, 2016). Stefanie Duguay notes that, because Tinder relies on Facebook as a kind of guarantor that users on the app are authentic, it 'benefits from Facebook fostering presentable users who abide by norms' (2017, 357), and it draws a direct line between authenticity and normativity in its marketing materials by emphasising young white heterosexual people (2017, 357–358). Kenneth Hanson (2021) has also found that app use among heterosexual college students reinforces whiteness and gendered norms. Even on apps that target LGBTQ+ users, such as Grindr, an app predominantly for gay men, heteronormativity is evident, with users often rejecting potential partners who do not fit a normative ideal, in that they might be 'older, black, short, fat, with long hair, and, mainly, …effeminate' (Saraiva et al., 2020, 127). Similarly, a study of bisexual women using Tinder in New Zealand found that these users were positioned 'as "outsiders" in a heteronormative and biphobic domain' (Pond & Farvid, 2017, 20). Indeed, as articulated later users who were practising sexually 'diverse' ways of living found both Tinder and Bumble limiting and binary at times.

The majority of participants who were heterosexual, and ascribed to a binary gender, often described specific milestones or occurrences which were required to trigger the romantic masterplot(s) (chiefly examined within this research), for example, the meet-cute, or the need for an important romantic story to be launched in a happenstance kind of a way, and this conflicted with their dating app usage.

The meet-cute

The meet-cute is a trope rooted particularly in filmic romantic comedies, where 'the prospective lovers encounter each other and sparks fly' (Grindon, 2011, 9). It is neatly meta-textually explained in the 2006 romantic comedy *The Holiday*, where Arthur (Eli Wallach) explains to Iris (Kate Winslet).

Participants consistently evoked the idea of the meet cute without necessarily using the words, for example:

> I always thought I would … my eyes would like meet his across a crowded room or something … or we would reach for the same croissant or you know something …

Importantly, the meet-cute is always accidental. Dating apps, therefore, which rely on a logic of active choice and not on happenstance, are not at all conducive to this kind of rom-com moment: as Thomas Doherty (2010, 26) writes, 'hooking up via match.com is *not* a meet cute' (emphasis in original). This leaves people seeking romance caught between two opposing forces. The apps provide their best opportunity to meet someone (especially during a global pandemic), but they also close down the possibility of the kind of romance they may have envisioned for themselves (usually envisioned in specifically narrative terms). Some participants felt an important romantic companion should be heralded by a meeting that could be framed as a story, and told to others in the future:

> My parents met at school – they were child-hood sweethearts, and my brother met his partner at work …. Where am I going to meet someone, on a dating app? What am I going to tell our kids, mum and dad met on a dating app … like, it's not a great story.

The gravitas of that first meeting in triggering the romantic masterplot(s) was described by many participants. This seemed to be a critical factor in emplotting oneself into a story of significance, and one that could add purpose and meaning to their lives.

In some instances, this led to a kind of roll-on effect in terms of self-confidence, where those participants felt like they were not special enough for a kind of highly narrativised romantic comedy moment like a meet-cute, and that the apps were their only option if they were to ever find a partner. There was a strong desire for romance to be 'organic', but also a strong sense that they were not the kind of person who could find romance without using the apps to explicitly seek it out. As one participant said,

> 'I'd love to meet someone on the bus, or in a café … and have one of those Hollywood moments, but I'm just not that type of person. I'm a bit awkward';
>
> and as another put it,
>
> 'Like, where am I going to meet someone? In the aisle at Woolies?'.

The opportunities for any kind of organic rom-com meet-cute were made even smaller by the pandemic. Here tension started for participants, many felt they were forced to use apps because no one was dating face-to-face anymore:

> Here's something else I'm angry about – friends don't set you up anymore. I don't know why – maybe they think there's too much risk involved. I have to use the dating apps. I don't like them, I hate them. But there is actually no other way to meet people anymore … like people don't just wander up to you and start chatting …

There was a frustration associated with dating app use – where participants didn't think dating apps could trigger the romantic master plot(s) required, however, there were no other avenues available for them to romantically connect with others. There was a sense that participants had been duped or had missed out on meeting someone back in the day when people actually met face to face, and this added to the Jagged Love anxiety which will later be described.

This didn't stop participants from acting strategically on dating apps. Whilst they described a need for a certain happenstance meeting, and invoked words like 'sterile' and 'strategic' in relation to dating apps – they acted in *these exact ways* to achieve outcomes. For example, participants talked about 'keeping their numbers high', meaning swiping left on multiple people, and keeping 5–10 matches locked in DM chats to achieve outcomes. They used phrases such as 'don't put all your eggs in one basket' in relation to not investing too much time in one match. This was indeed a reflection of Bauman's liquid modern, and the rolodex (in this case) of potential chat participants. However, ultimately, this worked against participants. In acting strategically, they appeared to confirm their fear that dating apps were sterile, and yes, strategic, and not locations for happenstance connections, or meet-cutes.

'The one' or 'Multiple Ones'

As previously indicated, the majority of participants were seeking a committed monogamous relationship via dating apps, and used their profiles on Tinder and Bumble to do so. Despite the media buzz relating to Tinder being a 'hook-up' app and Bumble being a 'relationship' app, the majority of participants thought they were essentially very similar, and for the most part, the same people had profiles on both apps.

However, participants seeking hook-ups at times have two separate profiles, or used two different apps – for example, one participant indicated he used Blendr for hook-ups, and Tinder/Bumble/Hinge for dating and relationships. A female participant indicated that she used Tinder for hook-ups, had crafted a highly sexualised profile (a series of images of her body, and the bio 'Here for a good time not a long time') and used Hinge for dating and relationships (with a different, more relationship-oriented profile). She said:

> I've always been really sexual, and I enjoy a hook-up. But I keep my eye on the prize.

By the 'prize' she was referring to the committed, romantic relationship. Echoed throughout the research was the notion that the monogamous-companionate relationship was the 'prize' or the 'gold standard'. Notably, participants who had the same profile on the same app for hook-ups and dates were MSM – indicating perhaps a greater fluidity in relationship narrative.

The majority of the participants didn't believe in notions of 'the one', but did evoke the concept, and did indicate that they thought there were 'multiple ones' with whom they could have a passionate, committed, relationship with – and this was a necessary part of their personal trajectory. The majority also indicated that they had previously believed in 'the one', and this was a result of watching movies, reading books and also role-modelled relationships – however, over time they had become jaded with the notion. One participant said:

> I used to believe in 'the one' and all that stuff … I watched too many Hollywood movies and thought that I would meet the girl next door or whatever – but now I don't think that's a thing … There are billions of people on the planet, people even have doppelgängers, so I don't think there is one person specifically there for me … but I do think there are people you get along with more, or are more connected to … or can actually talk to.

Rom-coms and literature were often evoked in discussions around romance and dating apps. Often to describe why participants believed themselves to be overly romantic. They seemed to form a basic template for what participants believed should occur in the dating app space, despite their derision of the often fantastical plot lines. The fact that they were often sited indicated that they were part of a collective psyche or understanding of romance.

Temporal and milestone anxieties – sex, and getting left behind

> I'm very close to my mum and she's a psychologist and I talk to her about almost everything and we often have a conversation about how I don't have someone in my life at the moment and generally I'm pretty cruisy about it, but sometimes I feel like the bite is a bit stronger … the anxiety around it is a bit more real … and she's a boomer, she's in her sixties, and she's like well why don't you just get on the dating apps, and I probably explained to you the same way I do to her, I feel like you can find intimacy on a dating app, but that's the exception not the rule. I'm a lot about the energy and if you're on there furiously scrolling, scrolling, scrolling, it's a must not a nice to have, I don't have any person is going to have a good experience with that.

Like this participant, the majority of participants described a certain temporal anxiety in terms of relationship milestones and life milestones. David Shumway (2003, 2) argues that we gain a lot of life lessons about romance from fictional representations of it. Importantly, this encompasses not just what romantic love is or what it feels like, but the constitutive events that make up a romantic narrative. As previously indicated when people look for romantic love, they are often seeking out ideas that they have imbibed from representations of love, or seeking to try and kickstart a romance narrative in which they can emplot themselves.

This is clearly evident in the interview data. For instance, all participants were quite philosophical and/or sad about never having met 'the one' or an equivalent to 'the one –' that is, the person with whom they can undertake those constitutive events of the romance narrative, the right person with whom they can achieve a happily ever after. This search for 'the one' sends them to dating apps. As one participant indicated:

> I'm turning 30 this year, and it's kind of that age when you start thinking, what does the next decade look like. All of my friends are now either

> engaged or married, some of them are onto their first kid, there is definitely more pressure from that perspective to take up dating apps more so.

This participant went onto indicate:

> There's definitely a sense that I've missed the boat …

This feeling of missed milestones was compounded by the pandemic, and participants reflected on this:

> I feel like Covid has set me back even further. Like it's going to be another year before I meet someone … maybe longer.

The timing of sex in relation to the masterplot(s) was also something that was reflected upon by participants. There was a sense that a hook-up couldn't lead to a romantic relationship, which is why participants looking for a hook-up but also a companionate relationship separated their two profiles. Hook-ups weren't frowned upon, in fact, they were seen by the majority of participants as a necessary part of life and relationships, however, not all participants thought hook-ups were for them, or often reflected that they had been there, done that and were now moving onto more committed relationships. They had evolved passed the hook-up stage of their life. One participant said:

> Yeah, I've been there, done that, in my twenties. I'm over it now. I don't want to go back there. I'm looking for something a bit more meaningful.

One participant set a hook-up strategy in place, where she hooked-up with 30 men across 30 days in a quest to feel empowered, and less invested in relationships.

> I just wanted to go back to that time where I was like fuck that … and just being like, bye, see you later, instead of crying over them.

The hook-ups could never progress any further, they had a strict purpose and there was no deviation. As one participant indicated:

> The first guy I hooked-up with was actually really nice. We chatted for a while afterwards on his balcony and I thought … he could be something … but that's not how hook-ups work. You're there for the hook-up, that's it.

The hook-up had very strict parameters and rules of engagement. Sometimes these were explicitly articulated by participants, particularly women. One woman said:

> I say when. I say who. I say how.

Another indicated that she often had the hook-ups at her place. When I inquired as to whether she was ever concerned for her safety given that she lived alone, she replied:

> Not really. I've never had someone you know ... breach the terms of our agreement, so to speak. The only time that sort of happened this guy turned up and he looked nothing like his pictures, and I was so not into it .... I ended up telling him he looking nothing like his pictures and he needed to go. He kind of begged a bit but then ended up leaving.

The hook-up, unlike the romantic connection, was incredibly pre-meditated. Details were discussed in advance in terms of locations, times and even sex styles. This conflicted with the discussions which related to romantic connections which tended to be high-level, minutiae, mundane chit-chat kind of stuff. For the latter, it was almost as though participants were waiting for the kind of magic required for a romantic connection, but were unwilling to be the first to inspire that sort of magic. Instead as Bauman described they came to belong to the mundane, chit-chat, the busy-ness of the dating apps, rather than the outcomes, the companionate love they sought. As Bauman writes:

> We belong to the even flow of words and unfinished sentences (abbreviated, to be sure, truncated to speed up the circulation). We belong to talking, not what talking is about ... Stop talking – and you are out. Silence equals exclusion.

Jagged love and Liquid Love

Dr Jodi McAlister and I titled the unique anxious predicament that ensued 'Jagged Love' – cyclical, episodic and anxious dating app behaviour. This involved downloading dating apps (sometimes multiple apps), vigorously swiping, matching, starting multiple chats (with low-level personal investment), becoming quickly bored or exhausted with the process and their matches, deleting the dating apps and then after approximately two weeks of experiencing fear of missing out (FOMO) and loneliness, re-downloading the apps. The cycle would then begin again and occurred on repeat for several months during the lockdown period. Many participants recognised this cycle to some degree, particularly the 'down time' and would talk about being 'on a break from dating apps'. However, they found it hard to pinpoint the reason for the loop, or the loop itself.

The cycle itself and the emotions experienced were heightened – high-highs and low-lows were described almost side-by-side. Participants detailed swings from extreme elation at having experienced a dating app connection, to utter ambivalence, and deletion of dating apps. There was nothing fluid about the shifts, the experiences reported seemed elevated and intense. One participant indicated, 'I've never cried this much before'. Similarly, there was nothing fluid about the relationship type participants were seeking, they were by no means liquid moderns, they acted as solid moderns during the pandemic.

There were several key factors that led participants from the high end of the jagged love cycle, as discussed above, to the low end, where they became disenchanted with the apps. One was the low level of investment in potential matches, which led to participants feeling bored and exhausted by their in-app interactions. Berlant (1998, pp. 282–283) argues that intimacy 'involves an aspiration for a narrative about something shared, a story about both oneself and others that will turn out in a particular way'. This idea of 'sharing' is echoed by various scholars in relation to intimacy. McGlotten (2013, p. 1) indicates intimacy involves sharing something that is 'inward to our personhood'. Giddens (1991, 1992) describes the need for mutual self-disclosure, with which Jamieson (1998, p. 1) concurs, contending that intimacy is characterised by 'constantly revealing your inner thoughts and feelings to each other'. As participants sought to keep their 'numbers high' – often a strategy to ensure that at least one of the matches would 'come off', or a ploy to guard against 'obsessing over someone' – this mutual self-disclosure and sharing of intimate details required to form an intimacy did not occur. Instead, participants were stuck in what they described as 'boring' and often 'exhausting' and repetitive chats that involved colourless discussions and topline details about their lives. One participant indicated:

> I also hate the mundane chat, and I lose interest going through that phase of that small stuff. And it's fine when you're on a first date and you're face to face, because you can pick up on a vibe from them and have a joke … it's just really artificial online. It's like the middle level has been removed, and then the two levels on either side are still there. It's like that game with the shuffle board, like you're throwing it to them and they're throwing it back.

We see here that the dating app paradigm not only removes some the key milestones and signposts of the romance narrative (the in-person first date, for instance), but also the accompanying emotional context. One of the core narrative promises of romance is excitement or magic, but what participants are experiencing here is the opposite: boredom. This mundane, low-investment chat was a key factor for the deletion of dating apps. Participants lost faith that the dating app paradigm could provide them with the entry point to the romantic masterplot, and they found it very difficult to reach the level of communication required to build any kind of intimacy in the digital space of the app.

Participants also expressed the notion that once they returned to physical settings, love would once again have an opportunity to run its natural and 'organic' course. For instance, this participant stated:

> I probably feel more hopeful about the end of isolation. I think that the nature of online dating might slightly change, because people will be wanting to have more human contact, they'll want to be going out more and

> connecting … for me I'm thinking to that phase, and I'm happy to go through this stage now.

This idea that solely digital encounters were not sufficient to determine whether or not someone was a potential partner and that physical interaction was fundamentally manifested in several ways. First, participants became disenchanted with the lack of investment evident in DM conversation over multiple matches. But second, they were also reticent to 'over-invest' in one person, given they might not be able to meet this person face-to-face for an extended (and unknown) time period. Participants were concerned that they might 'over-invest' in a match and then discover that they had 'no chemistry' in a real-world environment. Participants often described an 'animated' quality that was lost on dating apps, a three-dimensional component that could not quite be transmitted in the digital landscape, constituting part of the potential 'chemistry'. For example, according to this participant:

> There's so much lost in the digital domain. It's kind of harsh, because there are key things about you that just don't come across. Like, are you polite to people? Do you have good posture? Are you a smiley person? Are you loud? Are you quiet? What if I meet them face to face and the chemistry is just not there?

There was often judgment directed towards those who had been in immersed in fully 'digital' romances, which lacked face-to-face components. A certain derision was cast towards these 'faux' types of relationships, such as by this participant:

> I've got a girlfriend at the moment who is six months into an online romance or telephone romance or video romance or whatever that is, but they haven't met yet. But unless you put it into the real world you just never, never know. You just don't. It can be this kind of Jane-Austen-esque life and romance, but if you don't have that chemistry, and that smell and that attraction in real life, it's just not going to translate.

Chemistry, here, is something ineffable that can only be ascertained in the physical realm. Catherine Belsey (1994, p. 23) argues that the promise of 'true love as the romances portray' is 'to bring mind and body back into perfect unity', uniting '[p]hysical sensation, the overwhelming intensity of erotic desire' with 'rational and moral commitment, a shared life of sympathy and support'. We could roughly equate these with 'chemistry' and 'intimacy'. Participants were frustrated at not being able to develop the latter in the app space, but do seem to have maintained a belief that it was possible, albeit a fluctuating belief depending on where they were in the jagged love cycle. The former, however, was positioned as impossible without a physical encounter. The pandemic provided no opportunities for these physical meetings to occur. This thus became one of the reasons – alongside the failure of the development of intimacy – that participants became bored and exhausted with the dating app process and the behaviours that app architecture engenders, such as multiple matches and low-level investment. For example, according to one participant:

> I actually don't know where any of this can go … I'm chatting to all of these people, but I can't physically meet them, so maybe I'm just talking to them out of boredom. Like it's a little ping of excitement.

This represented the other end of the jagged love cycle, the initial excitement about the potential of finding an iso-partner followed by a despair about the possibility of romance being possible in such an environment. However, participants soon cycled back. The majority spent a couple of weeks off app before re-downloading, expressing a sense of FOMO or loneliness as a key driver for this. We use the specific term FOMO here, as participants defined a clear FOMO, an idea that 'everyone is on the apps' and that if they weren't participating in this paradigm they had essentially 'committed relationship suicide'.

The cyclical use of dating apps is not a new phenomenon. The drift of users on and off apps is often driven as much by dissatisfaction as it is by users finding a secure and lasting romantic relationship. However, in the heightened circumstances of the pandemic, the fluidity of this process – its liquid nature, to use Bauman's (2003) terms – disappeared. There was nothing fluid about going from maniacally swiping and chatting, deleting, to returning to the apps, nor about what they were seeking. Participants were clearly rattled by the jagged cycle, expressing in a consistent sense that they were personally 'broken' or there was 'something wrong with [them]'. The pandemic saw a desperation from participants to emplot themselves in the romance masterplot, to attain the security that provides, to not miss their 'right' moment for love, and an excitement about the unique affordances of the lockdown for a particular kind of romantic narrative. However, it also saw despair about the difficulties of proceeding beyond small talk to more intimate levels of conversation, and the inability to determine romantic chemistry without physically meeting. Trapped in the jagged love cycle, participants found themselves both strongly desiring romance, but unable to reach the apotheosis of the romantic masterplot.

Bauman and busy-ness

However, what held firm within Bauman's Liquid Love theory was the concept of busy-ness. Bauman speaks of how we come to belong to busy-ness of our lives, the endless consumption of things and this case relationships. While the aim might be to connect or to relate, what comes to transpire is simply a busy-ness, an endless consumption of things and people. Bauman draws on Italo Calvino's, Invisible Cities, where the residents of Leonia, would say, if asked, that their passion is 'the enjoyment of new and different things'. Indeed, each morning they 'wear brand-new clothing, take from the latest model refrigerator still unopened tins, listening to the last-minute jingles from the most up-to-date radio'. But each morning 'the remains of yesterday's Leonia await the garbage truck' and one is right to wonder whether the Leonians' true passion is not instead 'the joy of expelling, discarding, cleansing themselves of a recurrent impurity'. Otherwise, why would street cleaners be 'welcomed like angels', even if their mission is 'surrounded by respectful silence'? What he is asking the reader is – are not the residents of our liquid modern world, just like the residents of Leonia, worrying about one thing while speaking of another? Are not the liquid moderns simply imbibing relationships one after the other in an endless cycle, becoming hooked on the consumption and busy-ness rather than the freedom the liquid modern should produce?

Here, there was truth, as participants described their dating app experience often as: busy. A frenetic kind of downloading of apps, swiping, direct messaging and ultimately deletion. One participant indicated:

> It sometimes feels like a job … and if I go offline for a bit and go back on, then there are like hundreds of messages from people. It feels like a full inbox after a holiday. I just can't deal with it.

This anxiety as a result of the busy-ness was echoed by other participants. One said:

> I see the little dots when someone is writing back and I literally get anxious, because I know I have to respond and I haven't even gotten the message yet.

However, this busy-ness was seemingly self-induced. Participants seemed to replace the reality of their office jobs, with other stuff, and chiefly on this occasion, with the busy-ness of the dating apps. And whilst, they indicated they sought the solidity or the certainty of the romantic masterplot, they came to belong uniquely to the busy-ness of the dating app. This seemed to contribute to the FOMO they experienced if they were off app. They missed the constant activity, as though the activity came to constitute something – maybe not a life milestone per se, but *something*.

Opportunities for reconfiguring relationship narratives

Not all participants sought a romantic-monogamous relationship on dating apps. Two participants were consensually non-monogamous and married and used dating apps to hook-up. Yet both indicated that Tinder and Bumble weren't suited to sexual fluidity, to consensually non-monogamous relationships of polygamy, and despite the fact that they had both made it clear in their profile that they were currently in a consensually non-monogamous relationship and looking just for a hook-up, their matches would often not read this descriptor, and would swiftly unlatch them following a DM discussion of this nature. Both indicated that apps like match.com were more suited to their relationship fluidity and that Tinder and Bumble tended towards more traditional relationship constructs. Several participants used dating apps for hook-ups, and some even discussed using dating apps to meet new people, or to connect, and even to alleviate boredom.

One participant indicated that she first started using dating apps when she moved to Sydney from Melbourne and wanted to meet new people, and also get a sense of the city. Dating apps gave her an opportunity to go to different restaurants, theatres and parks on 'dates' and get her bearings.

Many participants also used dating apps to simply connect with other people, or waste time. It was a source of conversation and connection, for example, one participant indicated:

> I use the online dating apps to have something going on, to be dating … but I don't treat it as the platform to meet "the one" and still in my mind I assume that that person I will meet them in real life. So they're almost a bit of a time waster, you're bored, you sit at home and you can start messaging someone… it's good in that sense, when you've got nothing going on, you can start a conversation with someone…
>
> For me, I'm just a bit old fashioned in that sense, I like to think of two people meeting in a crowded room, and I know that I should think of online dating as the virtual bar, or the modern equivalent, but it's hard of me to let go of that. Especially because I've read a lot and watched a lot of movies and I feel like … in a fantasy world a little.

There was some crossover here between the desire for connection, or boredom alleviation and the quest for constant busy-ness, the need to be doing something, or to be participating in the dating app merry-go-round that everyone seemed to be on at the time. Many participants echoed this sentiment of 'not taking dating apps seriously', and apps merely being an avenue to pass the time. Often this was reflected within the above sort of context – that a meaningful companionate relationship should be located face-to-face, IRL. Notably, Tinder has predicted that the world of online dating will lean more towards connection, and less towards hook-ups and relationships in the future.

Conclusions

Participants, the majority of which were heterosexual and ascribed to a binary description of gender sought monogamous, companionate relationships during the COVID-19 pandemic via dating apps. In addition, they often mobilised relationship narratives in describing their dating app usage, and what they were looking for in a relationship. For example, participants often described the narrative 'meet-cute', or the concept of 'the one' and leant heavily on references to

Hollywood rom-coms, to provide background to their romanticism. At times, it was to deride the notion of the Hollywood rom-com, or fantastical ideas around the one, however, it was indicative that these tropes were often used as reference in relation to modern dating. Participants within this sample were categorised by a certain anxious-monogamous search, which I came to term as 'jagged love' in reference to Bauman's 'Liquid Love'. Bauman contends that relationships have become more fluid, where people are consistently looking for the next best thing, and that dating apps in particular, follow this formula, offering a new match at every swipe. This is all part of the process of consumption, of imbibing new lovers and relationships, the busy-ness of this activity being the critical functionality. The distraction. This was true and non-true for users within this sample. They weren't liquid-moderns, in fact, they were solid-moderns, seeking long lasting, monogamous relationships during COVID-19, perhaps to counteract the uncertainty of this period of time, where milestones and routines were stripped out of ordinary, everyday live, and replaced by a time-accordion. For participants, the relationship milestone was one that could be met during COVID-19, particularly given the availability of the dating app paradigm. However, at the same time, dating apps didn't offer the type of entry to the romantic masterplot(s) in which they took solace, they were 'strategic' and even 'sterile'. They didn't offer the 'meet-cute' or the IRL meeting they were acculturated too – which created conflict for users. Notably, participants acted in strategic ways on dating apps, despite the fact this was a turn-off for themselves and for others from a relationship perspective. The Jagged Love cycle was categorised by frenetic downloading, swiping, direct messaging and then exhaustion, boredom and finally a deletion of the dating app, only to return within a short period, in what seemed like an endless loop. Participants seemed to be addicted to the busy-ness of dating app usage, which seemed to hold firm to Bauman's hypothesis. Ultimately there seemed to be two layers to this busy-ness – a focus on participating and being part of the cycle, but also simply for connection. In a time of extreme loneliness, dating apps provided a space to connect, whether it was romantic, or ultimately irrelevant. Dating apps during COVID-19 appeared to serve multiple purposes: a conduit for meaningful relationships, an outlet for boredom, a busy-ness, a replacement for the ordinary daily routines that had been removed, a source of woe and a source of joy – making them a melange of disordinate things.

4

(DIGITAL) INTIMACY VS IRL INTIMACY AND WHY THE DISTINCTION *STILL* NEEDS TO BE MADE

Intimacy for many scholars is ineffable, unquantifiable and even ephemeral (Berlant, McGlotten and Giddens). Yet at the same time and for the *same scholars*, intimacy is connected and defined by the institutions, ideologies and desires that organise people's worlds. For example, for Berlant intimacy is entangled with stories of citizenship, capitalism, aesthetic forms and the writing of history (1998). To further complicate the definition of intimacy – intimacy is not necessarily synonymous with a private relationship, with love, sex, family or even friendship – and yet we tend to link these things together. For many people, to have a meaningful relationship (of any sort) is to similarly have an intimate relationship. But the core ingredients of an intimacy are ever-shifting. Can two people who have had a hook-up have had a meaningful intimacy? They might have shared their bodies, fleetingly, but not their minds, dreams or, even possibly, their names. Yet, this notion of sharing whether it is physical, mental or spiritual is present in the majority of definitions of intimacy. For example, Berlant (1998, 282–283) argues that intimacy 'involves an aspiration for a narrative about something shared, a story about both oneself and others that will turn out in a particular way'. This idea of 'sharing' is echoed by various scholars in relation to intimacy. McGlotten (2013, 1) indicates intimacy involves sharing something that is 'inward to our personhood'. This sharing is a deep sharing, one which includes reciprocity, and even vulnerability. As one participant described when asked what intimacy meant, 'It's showing another person how fucked up you really are'. It's an un-burdening of the soul, a sharing of our deepest and darkest feelings and even the sides of ourselves which are rarely revealed to others. Giddens (1991, 1992) describes the need for mutual self-disclosure, with which Jamieson (1998, 1) concurs, contending that intimacy is characterised by 'constantly revealing your inner thoughts and feelings to each other'.

DOI: 10.4324/9781003120353-4

Within the dating app context, intimacy is further complicated by ideas of 'digital intimacy', particularly relevant during pandemic times when digital intimacy became the only way to meet a romantic interest, or in some cases, the only way to facilitate a relationship. With COVID times compressing critical life milestones, intimacy, in the digital environment had to be escalated quickly, however, failed to meet the romantic narratives many expected. The modern world contains many forms of digital intimacy, for example, nudes, online sex and of course, dating apps. As social media, and dating apps, increasingly open up intimate lives and everyday social and identity-making practices to public and semi-public gazes, we are in the midst of important cultural contestations over the meaning of intimacy in the digital age. How intimacy plays out in the digital has become a prominent concern in the scholarship of digital cultures, as well as in a broader public debate. Intimacy is generally understood to do with the 'personal' and with 'sharing'. However as Berlant (1998) contends, intimacy is also socially and culturally constructed and sanctioned, defined by institutions, laws and social and cultural norms and practices. This now happens centrally through digital media platforms and dating apps. Practices of intimacy and sociality via the digital are increasingly seen as vital to the economically productive use of social media, especially for cultural intermediaries, influencers and other internet celebrities. Take for example recent trends around 'soft-launching' and 'hard-launching' relationships on social media – a trend commenced by celebrities such as Machine Gun Kelly and Megan Fox. The language of public relations, and digital public relations, has become enmeshed with relationships, love, intimacy and the digital world.

Simultaneously, many forms of intimacy and communication are being encoded, aggregated, analysed and commercialised, provoking unsettling questions about new forms of surveillance, influence and control, as well as distinct lack of transparency around new avenues of data collection tracking practices, and forms of governance. And while the latter part of this discussion is less a concern for this research it is important to acknowledge.

As a contemporary source in Cosmopolitan magazine suggests (2021), particularly in reference to COVID and iso-partners,

> Whether online or in person, and regardless of the level of additional information we receive (by looking at someone's social media, for example), in order to develop intimacy we still have to go through the process of building trust, communicating authentically, committing to the relationship, balancing autonomy with inter-dependence and knowing ourselves and our partner sexually.

It was this particular idea of 'getting to know' someone or the sharing required to get to know someone, which was a point of contention for many participants. It was the sense of the negotiation required to develop this intimacy, and indeed, the elements that were missing which included: movement, animation and investment. These missing elements came to block the development of an intimacy and went towards creating the jagged love cycle – the desire to find an intimacy but being stymied, both from a romantic narrative context, but also because of the limitations and compressions of the digital domain. There was a labour involved here, in developing this intimacy. A tension between devoting too much time to dating apps, juxtaposed against an unwillingness to overshare or overcommit to one person and to an intimacy that was forged only in the digital domain. As Jamieson (1998) would contend, there are face-to-face elements (or personal contact) required to build the intimacy.

In discussing digitally mediated intimacy, Jamieson describes the pessimists and the optimists in the nineties. He writes:

> The optimists in debate then, exemplified by Anthony Giddens, saw personal relationships as becoming more intense and democratically collaborative projects as people sought to anchor themselves through intimacy in rapidly changing worlds. For the pessimists, then exemplified by Zygmunt Bauman and Ulrich Beck, the same forces of rapid change were corrosive of personal relationships and rendered intimacy insipid, vapid and unworkably fragile. Exaggeratedly optimistic and pessimistic postures also haunt discussions of digital technologies and everyday personal lives, similarly implicating theories of selfhood and social change.

As Jamieson concludes the reality is probably somewhere in-between and not so polarised. The majority of participants were unable to develop an intimacy because of missing ingredients, chiefly the face-to-face component. However, others were able to develop deep bonds. For most there was distinction between a digital intimacy and an intimacy forged In Real Life (IRL).

The distinction between digital intimacy and an intimacy as generally understood was one that I initially sort not to make within this research. Given the ubiquity of dating apps and the interrelationship between the digital and our everyday lives, the separation between the two, seemed to be, frankly, outdated. For example, Elie Seidman, then CEO of Tinder, indicated on the Verve (2020) that younger people no longer referred to the acronym IRL, as there was no clear distinction between online and IRL – the two were heavily entangled if not meshed together. This is indeed a bold claim. Given that Tinder reaches 193 of 195 and has recorded over 65 matches worldwide (2021), their understanding of our intimate lives is at least noteworthy.

I contend, in this chapter, that a face-to-face quality was required for the majority of participants. Three key barriers were articulated by participants, a lack of: animation, movement and sharing – all of which, would have been alleviated with in-person contact. This is not true of all participants, some of which were able to develop significant relationships in the online environment. However, for the majority, what occurred in the computer-mediated space resulted in frail relationships, which could be easily disregarded and forgotten, exacerbating the jagged love cycle.

'Animare' – an overarching sense that something was missed in the digital domain

Jamieson (2013) theorises the self and the need for face-to-face contact in developing personal relationships. He writes:

> Face-to-face interaction and personal relationships have a privileged place in various strands of psychology and in the ontology and epistemology of the traditions of symbolic interactionism (Mead 1934) and phenomenology (Schutz 1932); intense, face-to-face, sustained communicative interactions are productive of a sense of self with agency and autonomy, as well as of a sense of a normatively ordered social world in which the self is anchored. In Mead, it is the interaction with embodied others in childhood which produces an inner dialogue with a 'generalised other'. The significance of physical and emotional interaction for the well-being of children and the significance of enduring ontological security are widely accepted within social science and are evidenced within psychology; people suffer long-term damage if their childhood lacks one or more loving relationships providing physical contact and attentive care. (Ontological security is used here to mean security of the sense of self and confidence in the continuity of one's being-in- the-world. The term was most famously first used in sociology by Giddens (1984), who drew on the fields of psychiatry and psychoanalytic psychology, particularly Erikson (1963) and Sullivan (1955). It was a key concept for Laing (1960), and also briefly cited by Giddens, whose sociological contribution was recently reappraised by Scott and Thorpe (2006).) Many contemporary social scientists writing about either subjectivity or personal life or both continue to draw on psychoanalytic psychology, symbolic interactionism and phenomenology, albeit eclectically and not exclusively. Over the decades, their basic insights have been elaborated or supplemented by other approaches more attentive to issues of gender, power and inequality. Proximate, sustained, emotionally charged relationships with co-resident or frequently co-present family and friends continue to loom large theoretically in some strands of contemporary theorising as the most 'significant others' shaping a sense of self, particularly in childhood, with other voices relegated to the background chorus (Berger and Luckmann 1966). If personal relationships are increasingly digitally mediated, is it simply assumptions of co-presence that need to be modified or does this indicate the need to theoretically uncouple self-formation and face-to-face personal relationships?

This final question relating to the uncoupling of self-formation and face-to-face personal relationships seemed particularly relevant to participants – many of which thought they simply didn't translate within the digital domain. They described a certain ephemeral quality that was missing in the dating app space. This statement from a participant encapsulates the sense of 'missing':

> I just don't translate into the dating app space.

This was common to the majority of participants, who felt their sense of self couldn't be converted into a series of images and a bio. There was something hollow about profiles, or one-dimensional. It was almost as though critical elements of embodiment, or personality, even of spirit, couldn't be mirrored on Bumble on Tinder. For example:

> There's so much lost in the digital domain. It's kind of harsh, because there are key things about you that just don't come across. Like, are you polite to people? Do you have good posture? Are you a smiley person? Are you loud?

This participant continued:

> Like if I meet someone at a cafe or something … like I'm going to get a coffee, and I start chatting with a girl, we have a joke whatever, I'm almost certainly walking away with her number – but on a dating app, I'll make the same joke and get nowhere, because all of those other little prompts are lost.

It was almost as though participants were *flattened* in the dating app space, and this process of flattening made them similar, if not the same to the millions of other people on the dating app, making the process of differentiation almost impossible.

The word that best seemed to encapsulate what was missed was 'animation' – which derives from the Latin word 'animare'. Animare means two things – first, it describes the movement, and second, it suggests the process of breathing life into a thing to give it a soul. Dating apps seemed to lack both of these elements: pragmatically, the static elements of profiles seemed to flatten a persona, and second, there was an ephemeral quality that was missed, a 'spark' of sorts, which could be equated to the concept of a soul.

The lack of movement to profiles was described by several participants. One participant said:

> Have you heard of Tik Tok? … I much prefer connecting with people through Tik Tok. I have a better sense of who they are.

When I asked what it was about Tik Tok which worked for her from a dating perspective, she said:

> I don't know … it's like you can get a better sense of who they are – who their friends are, what they find funny, or interesting … I don't know, even the fact that they're moving makes it different. Like you get a better sense … of them.

Notably, the quality of movement was mentioned by this participant, as though through movement certain nuances about a person are conveyed which go towards creating a chemistry or an intimacy. When I asked this participant about how she connected with people she liked on Tik Tok, she responded that she would look up their handle on other social media platforms like Instagram, and then gather more information about the person, before sliding into their DMs. This sort of gathering of digital bread crumbs also went towards differentiating someone from the thousands of other profiles.

Participants often commented that profiles seemed to be all the same, like they blend into each other as a homogenous mass – even though the people were remarkably different. She said:

> You just flip passed .... Swipe, swipe, swipe .... It's like you get stuck in the swiping, because they all seem kinda the same. Then sometimes you go passed someone and you think ... oh he was good, but he's gone, because you were just swiping.

On Bumble and Tinder matches lost their humane quality, and became just another profile, and this was a barrier to creating an intimacy. As the participant above outlines, users got stuck in the machinations of the dating app, for example, the swiping, which seemed to reduce the humane elements of the people they were swiping passed. This was reflected in how participants started to adopt a kind of digital dialogue in relation to their dating app use, by referring to people as 'cards' in their 'stack'.

Participants reflected that there was a certain impersonal element on dating apps. For example, many participants indicated that they were more 'surface level' when it came to dating apps and that they would make arbitrary decisions on potential matches which they wouldn't make IRL. One participant said:

> I'm cut throat on dating apps .... If they're not six foot and ripped, I'm like, 'next!' But in real life I would never be like that.

Participants often referred to this separation in behaviours – that is, between 'real life' and the dating app. Mostly, they referred to how they would quickly dismiss matches, be rude, and more judgmental in the online space. The reasons around this tended to focus on their being no repercussions, but also because they hadn't ever developed a bond or an intimacy with the match, making the dismissal, easy. She said:

> I guess it's the app ... it's like all those other details are missing. The one's that make someone funny, or quirky ... so you kind of have to be surface level.

Curiously, participants could add video content to their dating app profiles, but most felt there was something 'weird' when people did that or made their profiles seem overly contrived. There was an artlessness that was required in creating the ideal profile, which needed to seem 'natural' or effortless, and these effortless profiles reflected the desired quality, that is, that matches weren't trying too hard.

When participants were asked to create their ideal app, and profile set up, the majority landed on a customisable profile page (the first seen and swiped right or left on). Most participants indicated that they would have preferred to see more pictures at first glance, as well as a short bio or quote. Interestingly, most also indicated a customisable background might help to convey someone's personality. Again, it was multiple 'bread crumbs' about a person which went towards a cumulative effect of animation, and it was this animation that ultimately helped create a chemistry or an intimacy. Overall, the face-to-face element investigated by Jamieson, as the requirement for both the development of the self and interpersonal relationships was missing here, and most definitely required. Without this animated/face-to-face component, participants developed surface-level relationships or interactions which were as Bauman would describe 'frail' and 'easily disregarded'. However, participants felt these tiny slights intensely, they weren't unhurt by others behaviours in the online environment. As one participant described, the lack of intimacy, and constant judgement was something akin to, 'death by a thousand paper cuts'.

Low-level investment

Both Giddens (1992) and Berlant (2007) discuss the need for sharing in developing an intimacy. This sharing for Giddens occurs in 'pure relationships'. Giddens used the term 'pure' because the sustainability of the relationship relies only on participants' willingness to continue because of their mutual pleasure therein. The elements of the definition do not, in themselves, privilege the physical co-presence of face-to-face relationships, which as discussed, appeared to be critical in developing the intimacy and in encouraging sharing. Jamieson (1998) discusses how:

> In relationships as they are lived, mutual disclosure is not the only way of establishing intimacy and may not always be a sufficient way to sustain an intimate relationship. Moreover, while distance relationships can be meaningful intimate relationships, co-presence is a more integral component of some ways in which people generate intimacy than 'disclosing intimacy', for example, spending time together, providing care through practical acts and demonstrating affection physically.

For many participants, the first barrier appeared to be the lack of animation on the dating app and the need for face-to-face interactions to develop an intimacy. The second barrier to intimacy was the low-level investment they brought to matches. Participants talked about keeping their 'numbers high' – often a strategy to ensure that at least one of the matches would 'come off', or a ploy to guard against 'obsessing over someone' – which meant they had to keep multiple discussion chats going at the same time. As a result, participants were stuck in what they described as 'boring' and often 'exhausting' and repetitive chats that involved colourless discussions and topline details about their lives. There was a tension here that participants often described the labour of participating on dating apps. They would describe it as a 'second job', for example, the constant responding to messages which was required, yet they wouldn't over-invest in one person. They would spread themselves lightly across multiple participants, maintaining a high-level exhausting business, and yet seek to not 'over-invest' in one person, which wasn't conducive to the development of intimacy. Notably, this labour and intentionality also worked counter-intuitively for participants who felt the application of strategic was not very romantic. One said:

> Sometimes I have to keep going over the same details about my life – what do I do, where do I live … this repetitive chit chat, and it's just exhausting.

It was almost as though participants understood the nuts and bolts that went towards creating an intimacy, but sped this up for the dating app domain. The regular negotiation practises that went towards creating an intimacy were put into hyper-drive, compounded by the dating app and by COVID-19 which compressed time and milestones accordion style. This mundane discussion meant that the colour and vibrancy required in the process of self-disclosure never actually happened. The content that would have animated a discussion wasn't included. There were limited opportunities to get to know someone in the digital domain, as DM discussions were often trite and standardised. As one participant said:

> Nobody ever says anything unexpected. It's always the boring, hey, how are you? stuff. The worst part is, I do the same thing! It's not like I'm saying anything interesting either!

Instead, participants sought to make their profiles interesting – the labour wasted on creating profiles, which were often not perused by their matches, or on speaking to multiple matches in a surface-level way. To many, the dating app architecture encouraged this kind of meagre chit-chat, indicating that the dating app environment created a kind of artificial discussion:

> I also hate the mundane chat, and I lose interest going through that phase of that small stuff. And it's fine when you're on a first date and you're face to face, because you can pick up on a vibe from them and have a joke … it's just really artificial online. It's like the middle level has been removed, and then the two levels on either side are still there. It's like that game with the shuffle board, like you're throwing it to them and they're throwing it back.

These multiple elements went towards this shallowness of sharing and boring dialogue, the first being that none of the matches were individualised, because they lacked an animated quality and became a number in the dating app game, rather than someone with quirks, dreams and even, feelings. The second was that participants were often talking to up to ten people at the same time, and this meant they had limited bandwidth to progress the discussion. The last that participants also acted in the spirit of self-preservation, always keeping a part of themselves concealed so as to avoid getting hurt. During the first focus group many reflected that they had been jaded by online dalliances previously, and this meant they adopted the mentality, 'once bitten, twice shy'. This went towards the jagged love cycle – the constant busy interaction, and the lack of deep sharing.

This was not true of all participants, some reflected that COVID-19 slowed down discussions and made some more generous in their dialogue, more invested in their matches lives and less judgmental. One participant said:

> I think people are asking more genuine questions online now – like they actually want to find out more about you.

However, this was not common, or across the board, and many felt that COVID-19 exacerbated the 'boring conversation' phenomenon. This was also because participants had no certainty around when it would end, and hence had concerns that they would spend three to six months talking to someone, or investing in someone, and then discover within five face-to-face minutes that there was no chemistry. As indicated:

> I'm worried I'm going to spend six months talking to someone, put all my eggs in one basket and then discover when I meet them that it's not right … it's hard to commit to a real conversation or getting to know someone when you don't know if you'll ever see them.

Consistent was this idea that solely digital encounters were not sufficient to determine whether or not someone was a potential partner and that physical interaction was fundamental. There was an intense and instrumental cost-benefit analysis going on, which was in stark contrast to discourses of romance – that is, participants weren't willing to invest, without a foreseeable outcome. This was consistent across multiple participants. One participant summarised this statement:

> What's the point of chatting to someone for months online? Like we don't know how long we're going to be in lockdown for … could be six months. What if I meet them face-to-face at the end, and there's no chemistry? It's like I've wasted six months.

This is a particularly interesting quote, because while it reveals that the participant is sick of lockdown app-based dating, it also shows that their desire to find a partner has not abated. If anything, the uncertainty provoked by the pandemic intensified participants' desires to 'lock down an iso-partner', but chemistry could also be experienced via a face-to-face meeting, and in turn, this meant a failure to invest, share and connect online.

This lack of investment from people, this desire to arrest the development of any personal sharing, worked counter-intuitively, blocking intimacy, but also connection of any sort in the online domain – particularly during a period of time (COVID-19) where connection was deeply sought. Notably, this wasn't true of all individuals, but the majority.

The anomalies – those who invested in different ways

The outliers within this group were those who had developed an intimacy within the online domain, during COVID-19, or slightly prior. The interesting element to both of these experiences was that the people involved had not only fallen in love in the digital domain, but also *loved too much*, and both felt this imagined, fantastical love, had somehow been generated or conflated within the digital space.

Jamieson positions intimacy as a relational quality that is created and maintained by individuals through practices of intimacy – both real and imagined. Whilst the dominant discourse in modernity on relationships (and obvious within this research) is that intimacy requires a face-to-face interaction to prove chemistry, it ignores the bond that can be developed in an ephemeral, disembodied environment. Iveta Jukane-Hobein examines intimacy in long-distance relationships, and how these bonds remain continuous, and identifies the role of imagination. Jukane-Hobein argues that imagination allows for the practising of four dimensions of intimacy: embodied, emotional, daily and imagined.[1] Similar, to Jukane-Holbein I argue that dating apps are fertile grounds for the imagination and as a result can foster an intensely experienced intimacy. The imagined is very much required given the flattening of personas that occurs in the digital space.

Two participants developed a digital intimacy without ever meeting the participant. There were common elements to how they developed this intimacy – and a critical one related to imagining the match. Imagining who they match might be, and to some degree, conferring likeable qualities on that person. Roxanne said:

> I met this one guy on a dating app, and he was like your quintessential tradie Aussie bloke – and we started chatting, and we just hit it off. I liked his humour, and we started chatting off line and stuff. We literally talked for a week before we went on a date. Like we were on messenger all day talking to each other about stuff that was going on and having a laugh .... I had butterflies in my stomach every time he sent me a message. I was you know ... that stupid, giddy, kind of a vibe.

Both participants considered their matches digital presences, for example, they 'stalked' their matches Instagram accounts. This seemed to add to their understanding of this person and provide that critical 'animation' quality, but also assist in the imagining. Not only did they confer qualities on their match, but they also started to imagine shared life trajectories, or who they would be as a couple. One said:

> I kind of thought there was something important between us. Like I started to imagine what our lives would be like together ... like how we would be this funny, silly couple.

Similar to this participant, the other connected with her match on Tinder, and started a digital romance.

> He had this really nice way about him. Like, for one, he was really involved. Like a lot of guys my age pretend they're not interested or are super vague, but he was into things. He would actually talk and ask questions.

This participant mentioned that over a period of a fortnight, she shared messages, stories, pictures and memes with this person, and started to really like him. She went onto say:

> When we went to coffee for the first time, I was so stressed. Because I was like, what if he's not what I'm expecting and I've built this all up in my head? But then I met him and he was exactly what I was expecting – like the way he spoke was kind of similar to how he wrote in messages. Like 100 percent what I had imagined.

An interesting element to this quote is the imagined component. The way the participant had built up this person in their mind based on the 'breadcrumbs' found on social media, and also DM discussions. The other participant also referred to this imagined quality, indicating:

> He was kind of this muso type with long hair. I knew he was my type .... I could imagine us going to festivals together.

This participant developed a digital intimacy, which was deeply felt. She even reflected that it might have been nicer to keep it in that space where everything was imagined, where the messiness of bodies and IRL communication was not involved.

Notably, both of these digital romances ended in heartache. The first participant was ghosted after her first date with the 'quintessential Aussie Tradie Bloke' and spent six months in a digital-IRL-pseudo-non-serious romance with the person she met online, only to discover that he had been seeing someone else. It would be easy to argue that both participants were of a more romantic and less cynical nature and were more willing to let themselves be transported in the digital space, or, equally that both 'invested' in their match and were willing to share more to connect with someone.

Other participants derided the idea of completely online intimacies:

> I've got a friend who is in this digital Jane-Austen relationship where they've never met. They've been doing it for about six months ... I dunno, seems weird to me. Like sometimes it all comes down to what they smell like ... what's it called, pheromones!

What Sam means by the word 'small' is there an animal-like quality to attraction. Something that needs to be conveyed by physical proximity. The sense that these participants had invested too much, too soon and in an environment where intimacies couldn't or shouldn't be developed (in their entirety) was obvious.

Conclusion: intimacy, animation, sharing and jagged love

The dating app space seemed to flatten people, and they simply became 'profiles', lacking the animation required to create chemistry or intimacy. This quality, which was missed, was the sum total of the quirks and other details which seemed to make up a person – the sound of their laughter, the way they walked or even the tone of their voice. Many indicated movement of sorts would have helped to animate profiles – however, they avoided uploading videos of themselves to their profile (as this was perceived as being too 'try- hard'). Some participants indicated that other platforms like Tik Tok or Instagram (or even LinkedIn) were more fruitful spaces for linking up with a potential match. They indicated this was because there was more information about the match in those spaces, which gave them the opportunity to understand or imagine who that person might be. Arguably, the other reason they might have thought Instagram, Tik Tok or LinkedIn were more fruitful spaces for a digital intimacy is because the intention of these platforms is not dating or relationships – this means the initial meeting fulfils the 'happenstance' quality required in the romantic masterplot(s). The dating app *intentional* element, appeared to work counter-intuitively. The requirement for elements like chemistry and an ineffable magic quality was required by participants – and the dating apps couldn't deliver this. Notably, this was not true of all participants, some of which did develop intimate connections in the dating app environment, but notably all of these ended in heartache.

It was clear that for the majority of participants there was an element of using apps out of boredom. There seemed to be a need to participate in the dating app busy-ness, even if this meant just swiping, and not interacting, or keeping up multiple surface-level discussions, which continues Bauman's theory on Liquid Love and busy-ness – that is, participants came to belong to the texts, the swiping, the participating in the dating app noise as opposed to making a lasting connection. However, notably, the incapacity to build intimacy in the dating app environment fed into the jagged love cycle, the anxiety, and ultimately the hate/deletion of dating apps – only to re-upload profiles in a short period of time. COVID, again, exacerbated these tensions, as participants worried about investing in one person, without the face-to-face proof that chemistry existed. In addition, the uncertainty around when the COVID lockdown might end made it further difficult for participants – would it be six weeks or twelve months? Here, many participants reflected on the labour of dating apps – the idea they had to spend too much time managing their romantic life online, and yet conversely this labour was pitched in the wrong direction. They spread themselves thin across multiple matches, coming to belong to the busy-ness of the app as opposed to investing in the one person.

Note

1 http://www.iiass.com/index.php?option=com_content&view=article&id=990

5

HIGH-MAINTENANCE GIRLS AND AUSSIE BLOKES

Love and gender stereotypes during COVID times

In this chapter, I examine the ways in which gender scripts can be negotiated, reinforced and/or subverted on dating apps, focusing primarily on heterosexual app-based dating in Australia. While there has been significant negative commentary about dating apps and concern expressed about the potential effects they could have on the emotional and sexual health of users and 'traditional' institutions such as marriage and monogamy (see, for example, Ng, 2019; Fetters & Tiffany, 2020), there is no denying that dating apps are now one of the central arenas in which people pursue relationships, ranging from short-term hookups to long-term romantic partnerships. As discussed earlier, romantic narratives still play a powerful role in how users negotiate and interact on dating apps. In discussing romantic narratives, the role of gender and gender scripts is fundamental.

This discussion is divided into two sections. The first deals with masculinity and the apps, the second with femininity. I outline how archetypes of masculinity such as the 'Aussie Bloke' emerged in surprising ways, as well as the concept of the 'High-Maintenance Girl'. Participants were aware of the gender scripts they adopted and even in some cases extended, however, seemed unable to shift the narrative. This worked in two ways, both in how participants described themselves via their profile, but also in how they interacted with their match. The 'Aussie Bloke' was incredibly problematic, particularly for an Australian queer man of Chinese-Malay descent who participated in the research. He described the othering which often occurred on dating apps, for example, 'No Asians. Just a preference'. This was also raised by other diverse participants, and curiously by white participants who also sought to portray themselves in this modernised version of the Larrikin, but found it slippery and difficult to embody. Whilst the 'Aussie Bloke' was discussed by many participants – women and men – it seemed

DOI: 10.4324/9781003120353-5

that none of the men felt that they were actually able to exemplify the label, and felt as a result, that they were consistently doing something wrong.

The 'Aussie Bloke' itself was an updated paradigm – as shall later be discussed. Modern-day ideas of the hipster (in particular the beard) were woven into other more traditional elements that you might consider within the 'Aussie Bloke' space like humour, and a muscular or strapping build. Leo, again, described how the 'Aussie Bloke' was assumed, but changed into a 'gay-Aussie-Bloke' kind of a way. Despite this re-posturing of the stereotype, it was clear that the idea seemed to typify an ideal way of male presentation on Tinder and Bumble.

However, gender stereotypes were also shifted in interesting and unexpected ways, for example, men in the sample were more anxious than women in relation to how they presented themselves. Their corporeality and embodiment of the 'Aussie Bloke' were critical to their dating app presentation – and often they used filters, and apps like 'FaceTune' to achieve the desired outcome. Women on the other hand were more focussed on portraying behavioural characteristics, via the representation of the non 'High-Maintenance Girl'. Comparatively, men were more concerned with their physical presentation, subverting traditional stereotypes in this space. Equally, women's profiles were less shaped by the 'male gaze', and men more so by the 'female gaze' – which I will seek to unpack in the comparative section within this chapter. Notions of erotic capital and heterosexiness were again reinforced and subverted – as participants mobilised different signs and symbols, which were received by their potential matches often in unexpected ways.

I would hypothesise that the leaning on archetypical gendered ways of being was impacted by COVID-19 (and the uncertainty of the period) – which saw participants cling to 'known' cultural ideals, and steer away from explorative relationship paradigms towards more traditional ways of living a relationship. It occurred to me that there was less potential room for exploration of gender scripts and ways of being given the uncertainty of the period. However, this is not to say that there was a homogenising effect on self-presentation, ways of being and negotiating relationship paradigms on dating apps. In fact, there was an anxiety to self-presentation and interactions, and a vulnerability, which led to a certain shakiness in participation, which all went towards the 'jagged love' cycle. Unlike Bauman's ideas of 'Liquid Love' where transitions are fluid, and transactions are quick and transactional, filled with ease, the representation of self on dating apps during COVID-19 and presentation of self was a source of great friction and difficulty. Participants struggled to embody ideals and felt they were constantly missing the mark. Again, the labour involved in self-representation was high, as participants heavily curated their profile to represent themselves in the 'right' way. This labour conflicted with the at times flippant and apathetic approach participants had to dating apps, creating tension. Participants struggled on which emotion to occupy, fixation, flippancy, anger, apathy, fear, joy and even, hopelessness, creating a jagged rotation of emotions.

Masculinity on dating apps: the 'Aussie Bloke'

One archetype of masculinity permeated the sample: the 'Aussie Bloke'. He was positioned as both an object of desire for some women seeking a male partner on the app, and as what the male users aspired to be. This gender script had certain distinct signifiers. The Aussie Bloke is muscular, drinks beer (but not too much), has mates, might have a beard, and is tanned, tall and funny. Leo expressed it quite succinctly: 'You've got facial hair, you drink beer, you work out'. Another participant said:

> ...I like Aussie men... I much prefer Australian men. [...] I definitely feel like I need a taller man. So men that are a little bit more rugged, that have a beard or a hairy chest and I think as well guys that I can see have a sense of humour. That's quite big for me. Guys that I can see laugh at themselves, and can take the piss out of themselves... Aussie guys, they're generally pretty good at that. That's generally what the Australian culture is like. In a nutshell that's probably what I go for.

Across the sample, a 'masculine' or 'masc' man was consistently positioned as desirable.[1] In notable contrast, terms like "feminine" were not discussed very much by women, and not at all by men. This 'masc' Aussie Bloke identity was an aspirational one, one which many men in the sample sought to consciously portray themselves as. Using a sexual scripting approach, we can extrapolate that this is the dominant cultural ideal for masculinity in Australian culture: the highly masculine Aussie Bloke is 'a portrayal of masculinity by which an Australian male may measure himself' (Bowers, 2017, 300). However, whilst there were recognisable elements from the traditional Aussie Bloke, this cultural ideal was also updated in an interesting 2020 kind of a way. Unsurprisingly, it was an ideal that many men in the sample found difficult to live up to.

The Aussie Bloke – the archetype and the updates

The Aussie Bloke is one of the most identifiable archetypes of Australian identity. Indeed, it may be *the* archetype of Australian identity: as Linzi Murrie argues, Australian identity is highly gendered and marked as inherently masculine (1998). Murrie offers a description of the archetype:

> Our man is practical rather than theoretical, he values physical prowess rather than intellectual capabilities, and he is good in a crisis but otherwise laid-back. He is common and earthy, so he is intolerant of affectation and cultural pretensions; he is no wowser, uninhibited in the pleasures of drinking, swearing and gambling; he is independent and egalitarian, and is a hater of authority and a 'knocker' of eminent people. This explicit rejection of individualism is echoed in his unswerving loyalty to his mates.
>
> *(1998, 68)*

The model of Australian masculinity has deep roots in Australian colonial history. It emerges in figures like the colonial frontiersman and the ANZAC,[2] persists in figures like the surf lifesaver and the sporting larrikin and is perpetuated nationally and internationally through popular culture (Waling, 2019, 7). These figures are part of what Murrie calls the 'Australian legend' when she argues that '[t]he Australian legend has been a powerful fiction for constructing and legitimising dominant meanings of "masculine" and "Australian" in Australian culture' (1998, 75).

As Catriona Elder notes, the Aussie Bloke is '[o]ne of the most stereotyped, out of date and yet long-lived and most popular narratives of Australian-ness' extant (2020, 2). It is a figure considered by many with irony, and yet its influence is still deeply felt, as its repeated invocation in the sample shows (Elder, 2020, 3). It is a hegemonic identity, bound up with patriarchy, whiteness, colonialism and heterosexuality. It is resisted by many – see, for instance, Karina J. Butera's study of 'neo-mateship', where she finds that Australian men are beginning to expand the parameters of typical gendered behaviours in their friendships (2008). It is also an identity that has historically not been terribly friendly towards women. Famously, Miriam Dixson argues in *The Real Matilda* that Australian society is one of the most misogynistic in the world, due in large part to the way that Australian culture mythologises hegemonically masculine men and mateship (1999). Similarly, Jack Bowers argues that when we read Australian identity through a masculinist lens, we can observe how it speaks for men – and silences women (2017, 300). This probably accounts for the fact that the desire for an Aussie Bloke was by no means universal for the heterosexual women in the sample. However, the immense emphasis that has historically been placed on this archetype of masculinity in Australian culture, it is perhaps unsurprising that he is repeatedly invoked in the sample and positioned as the figure that men want to be and that women want to be with.

One of the major ways the Aussie Bloke is imagined is through his physicality: he is rugged, he is muscular, and he is tanned. This was reflected strongly in the sample, where the male dating app profile, much more so than the female dating profile, was defined by physicality: in particular, muscles and tans. When asked how and why men had selected particular images for their profile, they were quick to describe them as staged, contrived or even altered in order to create a more 'masculine' representation of self. For example, some men within the sample indicated that they had used filters to drive a higher level of erotic capital, especially through a tan. For instance, Taj indicated, 'I've gotten really good at taking a nice selfie for the dating apps. I'll also use a filter, like the mocha one on SnapChat which makes me look really tanned'. Similarly, another participant (male, MSM, white, 30 years old, living in Parramatta) said, 'I use the photos that make me look more masculine. Muscles, tight shirt, that sort of thing… I'll FaceTune it if needed'. While this was clearly intended to be a display of hetero-sexiness, it did not necessarily work on the women seeking male partners on the apps, who routinely found things like gym photos showing off abs or photos of a man surrounded by beers to be 'strange', 'toxic' and/or 'narcissistic'. However, these photos were deliberately included by male participants as a way of proving their masculinity: for example, three male participants noted that they had deliberately included shirtless photos of their abs for this reason, in an effort to raise erotic capital.

However, an emerging characteristic, and one which was referenced by the majority of the participants, was the presence of facial and body hair, which was an embodiment of masculinity. The meaning of the beard or facial hair has shifted over time – whilst iconic Australian figures like Ned Kelly sported the elongated and unkempt beard, the beard went out of fashion in relation to the Aussie Bloke identity for decades. As Cherine Fahd described (The Conversation, 2017), the beard could be the symbol of a terrorist or hipster, and often the differential between the two is both the shape and styling of the beard, and also the other characteristics of the person. She writes:

> The way someone looks – the size of their nose or the abundance of body or facial hair – is an amusing topic of dinner discussions in my Lebanese-Australian family. The topic that has dominated lately has been the 'look' of my two brothers. With big dark eyes, prominent noses, tattooed muscles and distinctive beards, their appearance has become an anxiety issue for my parents.
>
> In the hope of reforming their style choices my parents have repeatedly told them to "shave your beards off, you look like terrorists!" Their justification was all around them in the Western media: young Arabs with a beard equalled terrorist.

However, in contrast, Fahd continues to write:

> The contemporary male hipster is defined by his abundant designer beard, in the manner of a (well-groomed) lumberjack or Ned Kelly.

Fahd raises an important question in what is the cultural meaning of a beard. In this case, participants mobilised the beard as a sign of the 'Aussie Bloke' and this was often referenced side by side with the hairy chest. Their reference related to the contemporary male hipster described by Fahd above – it was an updated version of the Aussie Bloke. Previous version of the iconic Aussie Bloke, for example Paul Hogan (1970s), sported no facial or body hair - in contrast to the description of the Aussie Bloke provided in focus groups and interviews. Hence, the physique of the Aussie Bloke is ever shifting incorporating new cultural and social trends.

However, notably the bearded Aussie Bloke again seemed to highlight the othering nature of the updated ideal. When one participant referred to the bearded Aussie Bloke she wasn't referring to the description of Fahd's brothers, there was an implied whiteness to the dialogue. Fahd's study collects a sample of men who appear ethnically Arabic, and have a beard, including Lebanese, Italian and South-American men, noting that all men within the sample have similar physical characteristics despite having diverse ethnicities (for example, darker skin, more prominent noses, dark eyes, etc.). Hence, these characteristics combined with the beard no longer fell into the 'Aussie Bloke' category but a different one altogether. Similarly, ethnically Chinese-Malay Leo struggled to grow a beard or body hair, and again this was an othering characteristic in the online environment, as he found himself unable to participate in the bloke-ness required to embody masculinity. Similar to what Penny Rossiter finds in relation to the term bogan:

> ... that what happens around 'bogan' is as fleeting and labile as it is congealed and sticky.

The ideal of the Aussie Bloke was as slippery and shifting in the online domain, as it was sticky and othering.

Archetypically, the Aussie Bloke is strong but silent. He is physically dominant, but he does not talk much, especially about his feelings (which he might not even admit to having) (Murrie, 1998). It tracks, then, that in the sample, there was a strong need to evidence masculinity via corporeality. Some male participants indicated they were interested in demonstrating elements of their life or interests via their profile, such as an interest in travel or the beach. However, there was less of a focus on including images that demonstrated that they 'did stuff', and much more on this need to demonstrate their embodiment of this particular brand of hegemonic masculinity. This was not something that men in the sample necessarily *liked,* but it was clear that it was *felt.* Bumble and Tinder were particularly viewed as driving this economy of corporeality because of the Manichean good/bad image swipe functionality. One participant indicated that he preferred Hinge to dating apps like Bumble and Tinder because it provided more personal context and focused less on physicality:

> I think it [Hinge] prioritises a kind of, like, it helps people understand you a little bit more, because it has prompts. So people get to know a little bit more about you, rather than just having that visual straight up. I mean, I think if you're a really good-looking guy it might work for you... like if you're ripped or whatever. I'm more an acquired taste.

This is indicative of a broad trend across the sample: while many of the men aspired to portray themselves as Aussie Blokes, they overwhelmingly found it difficult to fit themselves into this dominant cultural script. It was an othering identity, one which was impossible to live up to. In some cases, this was for racialised reasons, due to the way the Aussie Bloke identity is intertwined with whiteness. As one participant indicated:

> Gay men want an Aussie bloke. It's racial stigmatism. So quite often guys will openly write no Asians, and you see that a fair bit and that does impact you after a while. It's very prevalent on Grindr and Tinder.

For this participant, racial stigmatisation on Grindr and Tinder was a major issue. He also went on to describe the impact this had on his sense of self-worth. He went onto say how Asian men within the queer community in Sydney were either isolated or unwanted or fetishised under the description of 'rice-queens', often by older white men. This behaviour was mirrored in the dating app domain, and often in more overt ways through blatant 'No Asian' descriptions in bios.

He indicated that he sought to create a masc. profile:

> I'll try to hide the flamboyant side of me. For example, I'll use photos where I'm not wearing a flamboyant shirt, or where my guns are out ... I'll try to sound not to sound to queer or girly in my bio ...

He went onto say that often this attempt to embody a concept of masculinity would leak into his behaviour when he met a match face-to-face or over the phone.

> I'll make sure my voice isn't too high-pitched, or I'll try not to laugh too much – or I'll suggest a blokey place to meet like the Tap House.

In his e-journal, he described how this sense of trying to embody masculinity, and even to some degree hide his Asian-ness or make himself more white-Asian had an impact on his sense of self-worth. He writes:

> It's coming up to Mardi Gras so I'll go onto the apps for a while – and then go off because they'll make me feel so shit about myself. I can't change being Asian ...

This idea of worthlessness and an exposed vulnerability as a result of dating apps and the unreachable concept of the Aussie Bloke was reflected across the sample. Men had the sense that they were doing something wrong on their profile, as manifested in a lack of matches, but were not quite sure what it was. This came to be expressed as worthlessness and/or an inability to properly perform masculinity. As one participant said, 'dating apps cut you down. Like, I used to think I was an okay looking guy – now not so much. I dunno... there's something I'm doing wrong'. Most male participants disliked the emphasis on hyper-masculine presentation they felt dating apps engendered because they found it so difficult to 'do', and felt that they might perform better in terms of raising erotic capital in a real-world scenario: as Nikesh said, 'If I'm on a dating app it's like crickets... but if I'm standing behind them on the coffee queue and start a conversation, then I might get their number'.

One other nuance that emerged was that, for male participants, there was a deep link between their own presentation and what they 'wanted to attract', which was not necessarily described by the female participants in the sample. For instance, he stated:

> It's not so much about how I want to present myself, it's more about who I'm going to draw in. Like, I'm not just after sex, the endgame is a relationship, so I don't want to seem like a fuckboi or anything. Like, I'm a bit of a sucker for romance and love and all that, but I always seem to fall for the wrong woman… […] I wanted to show that – I don't know, I wanted to sort of be a bit vulnerable, because… I want something more.

This desire to demonstrate vulnerability runs counter to the Aussie Bloke identity, who is anything but vulnerable. However, it also demonstrates something of an understanding that women might not necessarily find the stoicism, silence and anti-emotionalism of the Aussie Bloke appealing, especially in a long-term partner (something which is also demonstrated in a lot of Australian women's writing about romance, historical and contemporary – see McAlister & Teo, 2017; McAlister, 2018a, 2018b). While the efforts by men to corporeally perform Aussie Bloke-iness assume that this archetypal form of masculinity is heterosexy, that it is what women will find desirable, we can see here the idea that it might not be the foundation for a solid and lasting romantic relationship, and some problematising of this pervasive cultural script. By heterosexy, I'm referring to the use of sexualised heterosexual images (somewhat aligned with porn), which have crept into self-representation on social media.

Women within the sample commented that seeing men with their shirts off, flexing their abs or biceps was a turn-off. It was seen as 'narcissistic' and overly 'vain'. The appearance of beers within photographs also seemed to have a negative impact on women's understanding of their potential match. She said:

> I hate photos of men with their mates and beers. It feels kind of toxic.

This gap between what men perceived to be a representation of the 'Aussie Bloke' or heterosexy and women's understanding of toxic-masculinity was large. For example, one participant said:

> My trainer (Personal Trainer) had all these photos on his profile of him without his shirt and he was a success on the apps, so I started putting a couple of ab-photos in.

I asked him whether or not this use of 'ab-photos' had yielded results and he indicated that he had noticed more matches after inserting a couple of these images. This ran counter-intuitive to women's feedback in the groups which indicated that they found shirt-less men's pics 'toxic'. Taj was the only man in the sample who consulted another man on his profile (i.e. his personal trainer), the rest indicated that they relied on the number of matches they received as feedback on how their profile was tracking.

Toxic-masculinity was a key term used by women to describe men's profiles. There was an obvious tension here between men needing to perform a concept of masculinity but one that wasn't overly 'toxic' – it was a tight rope of sorts. As Grosjean, toxic masculinity can be 'characterised by violence, sexual assault, bullying in schools, opposition to sexual minority rights but also mental health problems and suicide'. The idea of the Aussie Bloke has often been steeped in notions of toxic masculinity, and men in the focus groups straddled the line with difficulty. It seemed that the cultural symbols which defined masculinity for men, like beers, and abs, often described something quite different to women. Here again, there was an anxiety for men in self-representation, a shakiness almost, which went towards the experience of 'jagged love' on dating apps. Men were unsure of the 'right' approach on dating apps and the result was often a sense that they had performed masculinity incorrectly, or that they were 'doing something wrong'. Making the dating app experience personally de-stabilising.

Femininity on dating apps: the 'High-Maintenance Girl'

The dominant script for men on dating apps reflected what they wanted to appear as. The inverse was true for women, echoing Sinikka Aapola, Marnina Gonick and Anita Harris's assertion that 'establishing oneself as being a particular kind of girl means negotiating with what one is not or does not want to be' (2005, 3). The dominant script for female participants in the sample was that they *did not* want to appear on the apps as a 'High-Maintenance Girl'.

Unlike the men in the sample, the women did not admit to altering the images on their dating profiles (though, of course, this did not mean they did not do it). However, they all indicated that they were very conscious of which images they selected when they were setting up their Bumble and/or Tinder profiles and the persona they wanted to project, referred to by many as their 'brand'. The notion of having a personal brand was used heavily by women, in contrast to men who never mentioned the concept of a brand. McRobbie (2009) argues that women and consumer culture have become heavily linked and that women come to define themselves through consumer products. Smith (2011), also argues that from a romantic narrative perspective, women are less represented through romantic gender narratives, but more so through consumer product, and draws on the popular book series Gossip Girl (which later inspired the series) as evidence. Indeed women in the sample had a strong sense they had to perform a brand. When I asked one participant if she had ever sent nudes, she said:

> Absolutely not! That's so off brand for me.

When I asked her what was off-brand for her in relation to sending nudes she couldn't quite quantify what it was:

I'm just not that type of girl …. I guess I'm more the smart, professional girl.

However, it was unclear as to why the smart, professional girl wouldn't send nudes. Because of the Manichean good/bad swipe functionality on both these apps, women wanted to ensure their profile was heterosexy, mobilising cultural codifiers associated with femininity so as to achieve match outcomes (often associated with a notion of brand). For many, this involved selecting images where they were 'done up' (for example, about to go out, with hair and makeup done), or more traditionally feminine images (for example, wearing a dress). Sandra Lee Bartky contends that as the links between normative femininity and things like chastity, domesticity and maternity begin to loosen, '[n]ormative femininity is coming to be centred more and more on woman's body… more precisely, its presumed heterosexuality and its appearance' (1988, 80). It makes sense, then, that for female participants, images of oneself were such a site of anxiety and intense management.

However, it was not simply a matter of looking pretty and exuding normative femininity. Female participants in the sample also felt the need to ensure that they did not come across as 'high-maintenance': they needed to seem 'relatable' and 'not intimidating'. One participant expressed the dilemma this way:

> My every day look is an oversized tee and very comfy clothes, but on my profile there's the festival picture where I'm obviously done up and there are two other photos where I'm with friends … I did feel the pressure where you should seem at least, look pretty, but at the same time you need to look relatable. So I guess at the same time, people aren't intimidated to approach you. There is that pressure that you need to look friendly enough, but pretty enough, but not too friendly at the same time. It's a weird line. There's definitely a different image that you need to present of yourself.

This kind of identity management, where women have to straddle an impossibly thin line, is nothing new. It is particularly pervasive for girls and young women: as Christine Griffin argues, '[g]irls and young women are generally represented as having (or being) too little or too much; as too fat or too thin, too clever or too stupid, too free or too restricted' (2004, 42). Here, the line is between heterosexiness and effortlessness. Female participants feel the urge to look pretty, but also not so pretty that they might scare prospective matches off, or suggest that said prettiness requires an immense amount of labour (which might then require a prospective male partner to perform labour).

In a study of young heterosexual women at a university in South Africa, Louise Vincent and Caryn McEwen suggest that:

> Not being viewed as 'high-maintenance' means not complaining, not demanding too much, not expressing needs, not having expectations for

> emotional openness or fulfilment – in effect, not making any of the demands which are the necessary requirements for intimacy based on relations of equality and mutuality.
>
> *(2004, 13)*

It would be somewhat hyperbolic that this was entirely true for the female participants in the sample – or at least, true to the same extent. However, there was a strong consciousness of the male gaze present across the sample, tied closely to the idea that being high-maintenance was an unattractive quality. When concepts like 'relatability' and 'intimidation' were invoked, it was with the male observer and his emotional responses in mind, prioritising his comfort. For instance, one participant said:

> Well, I'm definitely not a girly girl. I'm more of a tomboy. So I've tried to not make it just bikes and stuff. I've tried to make it more girly. I've struggled a bit with that though because I think a lot of men can be a bit intimidated by that.

This mirrors the way in which relatability has been described by Akane Kanai (2019): as 'an affective relation produced through labour that reflects a desirable notion of common experience to an unknown audience' (4). As Kanai goes on to argue, there is a critique of perfection (especially feminine perfection) in the notion of relatability, but it is still deeply invested in and entwined with standards of perfection (2019, 4), which may account for the ways in which female participants sought to balance heterosexiness (hegemonic feminine perfection) with not scaring away matches (being 'relatable' rather than 'intimidating').

In some cases, making a profile more relatable was framed as making it a more authentic representation of the self. One participant said:

> Tinder was all photos, so I would just pick photos where I naturally thought I looked the best in. And then I had a friend go through it (my profile), and they said you just don't come across as the person that you are, like you've got all these glamour photos, and all when you're dressed up nicely, and it gives off the wrong impression of you. People feel like you're very high-maintenance … and I looked back at it and I thought you don't want to come across in that sense. So then I put in lower key photos, when I'm not dressed up, full make-up and about to go out on the town.

However, heterosexiness could not be sacrificed on the altar of authenticity. A participant articulated, if one had to pick, prettiness trumped relatability:

> Obviously, I'm not the guy looking at the photos, you're always going to go for the girl that's prettier. Guys say they want someone relatable, but if you get two girls and one is in her trackies and the other one is more done-up,

> who are they really going to choose? The prettier one, sort of thing. She's kind of unrelatable though … a bit high-maintenance.

The two quotes illustrate another common theme that emerged in the sample: a strong emphasis on reading, constructing and surveilling women's profiles *by other women*, especially friends. It is in the eyes of the female participant in the second of the two quotes above that the pretty woman seems 'a bit high-maintenance', even as she assumes she will be more appealing to a man on the apps. Similarly, in the first one, it is the female participant's friend who tells her that people will feel like she is very high-maintenance and that she should include some more relatable content. This was a pattern across the sample and was a marked difference from the men. While men strategised and experienced anxiety over their profile, they did not report turning to other people to discuss it. Women, on the other hand, would frequently gauge the number of matches and likes they were receiving, and, if they were low, consult a friend or family member for advice on what they were doing wrong. The friend or family member would generally then advise them on how to better calibrate their profile, dialling up or down the heterosexiness or relatability as needed. This process is neatly summarised by a participant:

> [M]y profile was very much me and who I am. And I found when I was using it, as girls do, we sort of look at each other's profiles, and even my mum, who I'm very close too. I was like I want you to take a look at my profile, and she's forever telling me I want you to wear skirts or dresses more, so she said I think you should add a couple more photos where you look more feminine … and kind of being something I've toyed with my entire life. Do I just like be myself or do I give off an air of more femininity? How do I present myself?

Other female participants went as far as letting their friends write their bio for them – as one participant (female, heterosexual, white, 21 years old, living in Sydney) reported: 'I feel like the bio is this fine line, between sounding cool and quirky or just being kind of lame. So I let my friends do it – they know me better than I know myself sometimes'.

This kind of consultation was usually expressed by participants as a form of care. However, given the way that this consultation usually catered directly to the male gaze, prioritising attractiveness to that gaze or trying not to frighten it away by being too 'intimidating' or not being 'relatable' enough, it is clearly also a policing behaviour. Sexual scripts at the cultural and interpersonal levels are being mobilised here, with intrapsychic scripts – that is, what the individual in question might *actually* want – being largely deprioritised in favour of more hegemonic understandings of what might be appealing to the male gaze. This was complicated somewhat in instances where peers reportedly sought to help the dating app participant appear more like themselves – for example, Bek said, 'I let some of my friends have a look at my profile, and they were like … you're not this person at all …. And so I ended up changing it'. However, even in cases like these, the goal was usually 'relatability': a state of being that positioned the app participant firmly in relation to the wants and desires of a potential match (i.e. the person they needed to be relatable *to*).

This is an iteration of a phenomenon observed by Kanai (2017), who has described the mobilisation of affective-discursive knowledge in relation to women making themselves intelligible in the online forum, as well as the role of figures like the #BFF or #rideordiebitch in reinforcing these ideas. This creates a homogeneous loop of heteronormativity, policed at every angle. Kanai writes that figures like the best friend are 'defined through a relation of proximity' and constitute 'a mirror reflecting back a self with idealised feminine traits' (2017, 915). In the app context, this friend and/or trusted female source appeared not just in relation to profile policing, but at multiple points in the app journey. They provided solace if something went wrong (e.g. a ghosting), or interpretations of the actions of matches, as in this instance, she said:

> Sometimes something will go wrong, like that time that guy cancelled the date because someone had 'arrived' from the US – and I'll be like, that's it, I'm not contacting him any more. But then your friends will get involved and give you all sorts of interpretations on it… and I'm like maybe I should call him?

Interestingly, there was no real sense of competition between participants and other women on the apps. This could be explained by the fact that one cannot see the profiles of other women if one identifies as female and heterosexual – all the images one sees are of potential male matches. However, the same is true for men on the apps, who frequently did compare themselves to other men. For women, the point of reference for the dating app self was other women, but not competitively: it occurred within a space of peer guiding and solicited surveillance. The feminine self was configured and mobilised online through a lens of other women, with the interpersonal level of sexual scripting taking on a profound level of importance. The cultural affects relating to what might make a woman valuable within the dating app space were discussed by women as a form of bonding and even care, but this was clearly also a process of regulation and discipline. It is a clear example of what Alison Winch (2013) calls 'girlfriend culture', which ties together intimate friendship and regulation. As Winch notes, 'girlfriends are essential in enabling feminine normativity. Their intimate networks of comparison, feedback and motivation are necessary in controlling body image' (2013, 2). Here, Winch is writing about body image, but the same is true in the dating app space, where friends help friends put their best foot forward – where 'best' is equivalent to 'normatively feminine'.

Comparative analysis – confirming and subverting gender stereotypes and script on dating apps

Participants both confirmed and subverted gender stereotypes and scripts on dating apps. The appearance of the 'Aussie Bloke' as an important and attractive cultural ideal was unexpected. However, the parameters around the Aussie Bloke had notably shifted, there were characteristics that seemed to hark back to ideologies of the Larrikin, however, others had been updated, for example, the need for body hair and a beard was a new addition. An inflection from the metro hipster, which seemed to run counter to initial ideas of the Aussie Bloke being on nature and not of culture. The Aussie Bloke was summoned via corporeality, tanned, muscular and handsome – and men were open about how they would often enhance their images through filters, and even FaceTune to achieve the desired outcome. This ran counter to traditional gender notions that men don't care about their appearance and that the appearance and vanity are a women's domain. Here, men were more focussed on their appearance, and women on behavioural characteristics, that is being the non-high-maintenance girl. Whilst women held onto the concept of a personal brand, which confirmed notions described by McRobbie and women being defined by consumer capital, they were keen to define themselves as more than just a pretty girl, but as a woman who enjoyed sport, work and their social time. The need to represent themselves as a brand could be seen as encouraged by the app infrastructure, which allows for users to package up their persona into a series of images and a description. Seemingly, to counter issues such as a lack of movement and animation as described in the previous chapter, women instead mobilised nous in the brand space to create understandable concepts of who they might be. This also described an ongoing trend for PR-speak to enter the dialogue of romance and intimacy. As Illouz indicates, love and intimacy have always been bound with ideas of labour, consumption and the market economy; however, this linkage has become more pronounced in the nineteenth, twentieth and twenty-first centuries. This leaking of brand into the space of dating apps and intimacy continues this trend.

This might seem to confirm Bauman's ideas that computer-related dating creates a virtual buffet, a market of sorts, where people are constantly sampling potential relationships, but always returning to the dating app, looking for the next best thing. Reinforcing ideas that relationships and people are constantly replaceable, making the idea of long-term relationships fragile, if not impossible. Instead encouraging a fluidity in partners. However, this wasn't accurate. Participants described an ongoing anxiety in their self-presentation, a vulnerability even, a fear that they weren't (in particular) performing masculinity correctly, which created a sense of shakiness, a vulnerability on app usage.

This was more pronounced in women – who consistently raised the idea that they felt 'pretty shit' about dating apps. There was a sense of vulnerability exposed here for men, which ran counter to traditional gender norms of men being stoic, strong and unfeeling. Women on the other hand were more nonchalant about the dating app environment, again subverting stereotypes in this space.

Notably, women used other women as sounding boards for their dating app profiles. They discussed how they would often run their profile passed their female friends to make sure that they had struck the right tone, or described themselves accurately. This ran counter to ideas of expressing themselves through the male lens. And while an argument could be run that they were still performing through the male lens, or internalised patriarchy expressed through their female friends, for many the process of building their profile alongside their friends was one of care, humour and even of solidarity. Participants expressed how they would set up to their profile alongside friends while having a drink or dinner, and the process being an encouraging one. Alex, however, was hemmed in by her mother, in terms of needing to use more 'feminine' images, which for Alex reflected an in-accurate portrayal of self.

In contrast, Taj was the only man who asked a male friend for advice on his profile. The rest of the men took feedback from the number of matches or likes they received, and to some extent, they were seen through the female lens. However, often there was a confusion here, as the images that men thought women would find heterosexy (like abs-out) were the ones that women found toxic.

Men often equated their focus on their appearance to 'strategy' i.e. they were looking to be strategic about getting more matches. This was more aligned with gender stereotypes in that men, approached the idea of romance and love through a strategic lens, and with the intention of gaining the numerical advantage.

Both men and women walked a tight-rope in terms of self-representation. Men predominately had the sense that they were doing 'masculinity' incorrectly, that there was something wrong both about themselves, and in addition their profiles. Women on the other hand felt they navigated a line of being pretty or heterosexy, but not high-maintenance. Both seemed to wander these terrains with a level of uncertainty, which worked towards jagged love. This sense of being on the unstable ground in the romance/dating apps space. It encouraged the love/hate relationships with apps. As they could both be a source of joy (matches), validation and a time-passer, but could also plunge them into the depths of woe and anger (lack of matches, ghosting or inappropriate chats). The time period COVID-19, and the uncertainty of this period seemed to exacerbate this sense of shakiness, as romantic and narrative milestones were compressed, and participants felt like they needed to sure up a match, which seemed impossible both because they physically couldn't meet anyone (COVID lockdown) but also because they couldn't represent themselves accurately.

Conclusion: dating on the apps during COVID-19

The sexual scripting processes evident here on dating apps are not new ones. Aspirational figures like the Aussie Bloke and negative figures like the High-Maintenance Girl have been circulating in contemporary Australian culture for a long period of time, and if this research had been conducted during another time period, it is likely that many of the same anxieties and scripts would have been invoked.

However, the global COVID-19 pandemic intensified and crystallised many of the usual paradigms evident in dating apps as people were cast into a state of ontological uncertainty by the pandemic and the ensuing lockdowns. Elsewhere, I have discussed this in respect to participants' attitudes to romance, observing that while the patterns of dating app use for people during the pandemic were not enormously different than previously, these patterns were 'heightened and accelerated by the pandemic, as people desperately sought the certainty offered by the romantic masterplot. This caused what had hitherto been a relatively fluid cycle to become fragmented and frenetic: or, as we have put it, jagged' (Portolan & McAlister, 2021).

This need to employ encoded cultural codifiers and prompts in images also speaks to the highly visual nature of dating apps. Operating in a visual economy users needed to mobilise the known signs and symbols to enhance culturally sanctioned forms of femininity and masculinity to drive outcomes. Participants were conscious that other users were making split-second decisions on their profiles based on their opening image (in many cases) and for this reason needed to make the image highly legible and acculturated to an understanding of what was attractive within a heterosexual space. As Dobson would indicate in relation to MySpace, and young women, digital spaces engender the curation of certain visuals which are perceived to be 'hetero-sexy':

> by 'hetero-sexy' (a term discussed below) material I mean imagery, iconography, and decorations on the profiles that appear, in terms of aesthetics and the visual appearance of bodies, to reinforce current notions of feminine gender performativity as 'sexualised'

And whilst not necessarily 'sexualised' within the dating app paradigm (unless users were seeking a hook-up), notions of 'relationship heter-sexiness' were mobilised to generate interest within a highly visual economy. The cultural codifiers within the 'relationship hetero-sexiness' paradigm read as highly entrenched and othering Australian symbols synonymous with the Aussie Bloke and the not so High-Maintenance Girl – embodiments of the Australian cultural heterosexual narrative. This was evident of both heterosexual and queer participants. This level of gender performativity was often concerning for participants, who often had the sense that they weren't doing something 'right', or that they were misrepresenting themselves within the dating paradigm.

And whilst Berlant might discuss the 'porous landscape' of digital media and the opportunity for users to explore different gender roles, and scripts, this was not evident within this sample – where users rigidly held to gender scripts and representations.

In some ways, the pandemic did engendered creativity. Participants could not meet in person, and so they had to figure out new ways to date. Some participants enjoyed this. As one participant (female, heterosexual, white, 23 years old, living in Sydney) said:

> I was reading this thread, some chick met someone on Hinge, and he bought her a drink and pizza and went and sat outside of her apartment so they could FaceTime and eat together. I think that's cuter and more connection then going out to a bar. I think people are having to get more creative around it, and I think people are enjoying it.

Others, however, disagreed, and felt very negative towards the situation engendered by the pandemic. As another participant (male, heterosexual, white, 27 years old, living in Parramatta) said:

> But at the moment there's this uncertain period of time, where people can't meet in the traditional way, so, am I going to bother keeping this up for an indeterminate period of time. I feel like people are keen to talk to each other, but not super interested in committing.

Given the uncertainty of the period, it is perhaps unsurprising that the dominant cultural scripts of the Aussie Bloke and the High-Maintenance Girl were so heavily emphasised in the sample. In an extraordinary, uncertain time, people clung to the ordinary and the certain in these known models for performing gender.

However, alongside these evoked gender scripts, there was also a subversion. Men were more interested in the portrayal of their appearance than women and more willing to tamper with their images (through filters and FaceTune) to achieve the desired outcomes. Women were more focussed on behavioural characteristics and steering away from the High-Maintenance Girl. Indeed, there was a focus for women on personal brand, however, this brand was not just a reflection of consumer goods, but rather of behavioural characteristics (sporty, hard-working, music-lover, etc.). Women sought to convey a level of depth, whilst men focussed on appearance. Men were also intensely vulnerable in this space, looking to express their sensitivities in quiet ways, but also personally in relation to their performance on the app. No matches equalled the sense that they were losers, unattractive or worthless. Whilst women were more stoic on app. Again, subverting traditional gender stereotypes.

Overall, there was a sense of anxiety and vulnerability in portraying self on the apps. There was a labour involved here. A consistent monitoring and curating of profiles to ensure they struck the right note, which meant that labour, romance and intimacy became heavily intertwined.

Unlike Bauman's analysis of Liquid Love, there was nothing fluid about this experience. IT was heart wrenching for many, and in particular men, who came to see this as a reflection on themselves, on their lack of masculinity and overall of desirability. There was a vulnerability and anxiety which went towards creating the right profile, which build on jagged love, but was also exacerbated by COVID-19, which compressed time accordion style, and made participants feel like they should be reaching relationship milestones.

Notably, the Chinese-Malay participant reflected the casual racism experienced on dating apps. Something that he described as a common within the queer community in Sydney, as directed towards queer Asian men. However, this seemed to be felt even more intensely, particularly when presented with black and white words on profiles such as 'No Asians. Just a preference'. Leo was the only ethnically diverse, queer man within the sample, however, it is important to note that this study is not a numerical one, and his experience needs to be reflected and examined accurately, with further future study within this area required.

Notes

1 Participants used the terms 'masculine' and 'masc' almost interchangeably, with 'masc' generally positioned as a more updated, cool word.
2 Australian and New Zealand Army Corps. The ANZAC is a figure particularly heavily associated with the Battle of Gallipoli in 1915.

6

MESSINESS – THREE ANECDOTES

Three anecdotes

In August 2020, I started a podcast series called Slow Love with the production company Contento. Our aim was to document love during COVID times. At this stage, my in-field data collection was complete, however, I still had a number of questions that didn't fit into the size and scale of my PhD. One of them was – what happens to intimacies forged during the pandemic, post-lockdown? Were they just as enduring as relationships developed IRL and pre- COVID-19 times? One of the key findings in this research certainly was that COVID-19 and the use of dating apps didn't necessarily engender the right conditions for developing an intimacy. Whether it was the uncertainty of when a face-to-face meeting would be permitted, a lack of animation and movement, the lack of romantic narratives, the labour of self-presentation, or the jagged love cycle – intimacies for these participants were stymied.

The other reason I chose to start the podcast was the subject matter within this thesis was so important, and so timely – it seemed that for most participants the significance of connecting and creating an intimacy was paramount – particularly during a COVID world. The stories that participants shared with me were so passionate, intense and unabridged. They retold components of their intimate lives that I believe they had never told others. There were tears, and even, shame.

Shame about being ghosted. About having to use a dating app to develop an intimacy. About not having enough matches. About receiving or requesting nudes. About never having met a significant other. About wanting things that were perceived to be pedestrian, like a romantic other.

It struck me that most of the participants that came to the in-depth interviews came with a desire to be unburdened. I was almost like being a priest receiving confessors. Only I couldn't confer a pardon of any sort, or three hail Mary's in

DOI: 10.4324/9781003120353-6

penance. This didn't seem to matter, they came, simply to talk about love, sex and intimacy, and be listened too.

It occurred to me that the avenues to discuss such things are limited. In 2022, real discussions about intimacy are still lacking. The podcast presented as an avenue for people to provide their intimate stories in an unabridged fashion. Many chose to go under pseudonyms, others relished in detailing their secrets, and disclosing their identities.

In November 2020, the podcast went top five in the Australian podcast charts, after we handed over the mic to an escort. She took on the role of host and interviewed one of her clients. The interview was a view into the world of sex work during COVID-19. A topic that went mostly undiscussed by the media at the time. When news.com picked up on the podcast, we hit an all time record of number 4 on the charts, directly behind the Michelle Obama podcast.

We ran the Slow Love podcast for just under 12 months and concluded after we failed to secure funding. However, those involved in the project, concurred that it was an incredibly worthwhile one, which compiled COVID stories of intimacy, similar to the Berlin love letter archive (only on a smaller scale!)

However, in concluding this thesis – I wanted to share with you a story that was captured on the podcast, which seems to summarise this thesis, the shifts in intimacy during COVID-19, the casual racism of dating apps, the labour of self-presentation, romantic narratives, but also continues to the final question, what happened to intimacies forged during this curious period of time?

Anecdote one

Michael Zhang is an Australian man with a Chinese background. He lives in Melbourne, and his parents own a chain of bargain stores – similar to Top Dollar. Michael has been looking for love for some time – he is close to thirty, and it's his parents expectations and his own that he should meet someone and settle down. However, Michael's not completely convinced about the idea of 'settling down' and has progressive views which vary from wanting to find a wife and monogamous relationship, to entering an open relationship. He seems to fit between these ideas somewhat ambivalently. Michael used multiple apps including Tinder and Bumble. However, he thinks that these apps are made for 'white' audiences, and he indicates that it's well known within the Asian communities, that Asian men in particular don't do well on 'mainstream' apps. He has in the past laboured to create a more 'white' profile however eventually gave up. He notes, whilst Asian men have no market on dating apps, Asian women are often fetishised in the dating app space.

Michael starts using an 'Asian' romantic app called Tan during the pandemic, and he meets a woman of his age from a Filipino background. He has met her previously IRL, and this seems to speed up the intimacy between them. They meet discretely during COVID, and not long after they move in together. There are pragmatic reasons to this moving in. She was looking for a place – and he wanted the company during COVID-iso. Michael seems ambivalent about whether or not they're suited romantically. He concludes that they'll just have to 'wait and see'. He indicates that their relationship has gone through a compressor. He also muses that only a couple of months in, they find them seated in front of the television in their pyjamas at 10 am eating celery. The 'fun' stage of their relationship had been removed, replaced by the mundanity of a more mature relationship.

I ask him whether he thinks the relationship will last post-COVID lockdown. He says it's a good question. After a pause, he indicates that they'll likely need to re-test the relationship in a COVID-free world. He says that he has never seen his girlfriend in a social scene, and never introduced her face-to-face to his friends. He reflects that the dynamic between them is a COVID-lockdown-specific one, which might not work in the outside world. But he's willing to give it a go. There is, he says, something between them.

Post-COVID lockdown, I check in with Michael on a second podcast, and he has since broken up with his girlfriend. It simply didn't work out, he says. They rushed it during COVID and came to dislike each other and the routine they fell into. They didn't even get the chance to test the relationship on the other side, once COVID lockdown ended they went their separate ways.

The course of Michael's relationship seemed to summarise the COVID lockdown experience. The COVID accordion time compressor was present. Michael met his match online, but the relationship was accelerated as they previously knew each other, and also because there was a COVID lockdown/COVID-iso-partner factor. However, in moving in quickly, and settling into a mundane paradigm, the pair removed critical relationship milestones that can be expected in building a romantic relationship, for example, dinner dates, meeting the friends, meeting the family, etc. As previously indicated, Illouz (2013) argues that love has been colonised by consumption, and in the mid-twentieth century moved from the confines of private courting, to the public, consumer spaces of dinners, movies, etc. She also argues that these spaces are highly visible, and that love requires this visibility to indeed exist. Both of these elements were removed for Michael and his match, as well as the romantic milestones which we have come to learn are vital to the progression of participants' relationships within this research. It was almost as though these punctuations (milestones), and visibility, were even more required within the COVID world, where time was flattened, and life-inertia was experienced. The romantic milestones would have removed the sense that he was otherwise wasting time in this relationship.

Anecdote two

The second anecdote I wanted to draw on was the beginning of a new trend – soft and hard launching relationships online (mentioned in this book). In December 2021, I received a call from Triple J. They were looking to talk to someone within the digital intimacy space about the new phenomenon of celebs 'launching' relationships on Instagram. This refers to how celebs announce their relationship in an online environment, and how this has seeped into contemporary culture. Indeed, celebs launching relationships is nothing new, it would have been done in the days of Liz Taylor and Rock Hudson – a romantic announcement to whip the audience into a frenzy, and as a result drive popularity for the pair, their movies, etc. However, this new form of launching a relationship referred to the images uploaded onto an Instagram grid and the accompanying tagline. For example, celeb duo Machine Gun Kelly and Megan Fox hard launched their relationship with an image of them embracing and a caption which declared their love (considered a hard launch), whilst Travis Barker and Kourtney Kardashian debuted their romance with an image of their linked hands and an obscure reference to romance (a soft launch). These celeb couples continued to document every step of their romances, right through to their marriage proposals. The idea that Triple J wanted to me to explore, was how normal relationships, those involving ordinary people, were also being debuted in a similar way. Indeed, anyone who has an Instagram account would be privy to friends, acquaintances and strangers announcing their love stories, sometimes in cringe worthy ways. When did this become an acceptable and important part of dating?

Not only did I participate in the segment, but I also later wrote a piece in the Conversation on the phenomenon (February 2022). Several things struck me when investigating this topic. The first was that the language of public relations had entered the realm of love (like the reference to the brand by participants in describing their self-presentation on dating apps), and that love was an asset to be marketed, an indication that a critical milestone had been ticked off. Bek indicated that she had the sense that life hadn't really started until she met 'the one', and this sentiment seemed to be echoed in the popularity of the Instagram relationship launch. It was an indication that life was ready to head into gear for relationship participants. I wrote for The Conversation (February 2022):

Your romantic social stocks

> Use the Instagram-official blueprint correctly, and your social stocks will likely soar. Take as evidence Kourtney Kardashian's Instagram account which grew by 44 million in 2021 following her relationship Insta-reveal. Love is after all the most popular hashtag on Instagram.
>
> Cultural theorist Lauren Berlant reminds us that when we're told to "get a life", it usually refers to the need for a person to find an intimate relationship. The milestone of finding a life-partner, is indeed, seen as a critical one which continues to hold cultural and social relevance. When we narrativise our lives, there are a number of acceptable pathways available, and the romantic union is a highly recognisable one, which has developed a certain visual formula within the social media space.
>
> My own research into dating apps and intimacy demonstrate how users come to recognise these signs as an indicator that an important relationship has commenced.

Again, here there was a process to how a love story should unfold, as documented through Instagram. There was the declaration of love, heralded by the soft or hard launch, the documenting of key milestones like dinner and beach dates, meeting the family, and of course the all important proposal. There was a language that was used here too, commonalities between words, like 'She said yes', or 'marrying my best-friend'. There was a recognised love-Instagram formula, which was indeed no different to the formula which was expected by participants on dating apps. And there was the business of jagged love, the need to participate in the digital love paradigm, or be left out.

But what happens if a break-up occurs? Does one simply erase all the romantic images of their ex on social media? Hence, removing the breadcrumbs of a relationship? Critical to the celebrity relationship reveal is the declaration of 'the one' or 'the love of my life'. One can't have multiple loves, or ones, if this announcement has already been made. Hence the need for the strategic removal (or deletion) of the previous relationship milestones, making way for the next announcement.

Lastly, within this social dating paradigm, another trend identified in my research – labour. The labour of curating the perfect relationship announcement.

Anecdote three

In mid-2021, I was asked to speak at Studio 10 about my research. After the interview, I caught an Uber from Pyrmont to my home in Redfern. The driver, familiar with the pick-up location, asked me if I'd been a guest on the program, to which I'd responded, yes. He went onto ask, what I had spoken about, and I indicated, my research, which revolved around dating apps and intimacy. This I came to learn over the course of this thesis piqued people's interest, and they would quickly tell me their own experience, or, if they'd never been on a dating app, they would want me to give them a quick rundown of my findings, seemingly so all their worst dating app stereotypes could be confirmed.

In this case, the Uber driver told me that he had met his current girlfriend on a dating app. He went onto tell me that he had worked in the finance sector but been laid off during COVID-19 and had started driving Uber's as a way to make ends meet. He was also using Tinder during COVID-19, looking for a partner. He went onto remark that the majority of women on Tinder were really just looking for someone to look after them from a financial perspective. Having previously worked in a lucrative industry, he was conscious that he was an easy target for what he unabashedly described as 'gold diggers'.

He went onto say that one of the biggest turn-offs in the online space for him was the presence of too many designer handbags in photographs. If he saw multiple Louis Vuitton's he would swipe left, convinced that this was a 'high-maintenance' woman, looking for him to pay for his lifestyle.

He remarked that he was now seeing someone. That she was a model, but also very low maintenance. Easy going and relaxed, he continued.

As I left the Uber the conversation was asterisked and underlined in my mind, and I quickly sat down at my desk and transcribed it.

The reference to 'high-maintenance' echoed the discussion in focus groups and interviews, as well as the strange interplay between a woman needing to be pretty or beautiful (a model in this case) but low maintenance. Alongside this, there was a curious reference to the Louis Vuitton handbags, and the statement that the brand was synonymous with representations of 'high-maintenance'. This seemed to interestingly link up to McRobbie's notions of women described through brands and consumptions. To my Uber driver, this was indeed the case. Finally, there was the term 'gold diggers', which hadn't been used in my research, but for this man, was linked to being 'high-maintenance' and to designer or high-end brands. This was the first time that a sentiment around women being 'too expensive' had entered the picture, and I wondered how far this permeated into my own research. Were men not keen on 'high-maintenance' women because they feared paying for their lifestyle? And similarly, did women seek to present themselves as not high-maintenance because they were signalling that they weren't gold diggers? It hadn't yet occurred to me that this might be the case, and unfortunately, it was too late to answer these questions from a research perspective.

Why these three anecdotes to conclude?

The reason I sought to convey these three anecdotes which had previously gone undocumented and were not part of the original research in the conclusion was that they seemed to summarise love and digital dating in the times of COVID-19. COVID-19 both flattened time accordion style, but also removed critical milestones, which seemed essential in our life narratives. Creating a sense of life inertia, or that we were 'wasting time'. This idea of wasting time implies that there is a good way to spend time and a bad way to spend time. Good ways of spending time are chalked up to key milestones, like an education, buying a home, having a meaningful relationship, etc. As Berlant indicates (2007) and I quote in the Conversation article, 'get a life' implies that one needs to find a personal life, and that inherently means a relationship.

The capacity to reach the milestone of the intimate other was still open to participants during COVID-19, but only through the dating app paradigm – another space that removed critical relationship milestones. For Michael, things were simpler, he was able to find someone on the app that he recognised. She stood out from the crowd, propelling him forward into a world of iso-partnership, which had it's own drawbacks (and lack of milestones), for others the lack of face-to-face contact, animation, and failure to meet romantic narratives, spun them into the jagged love cycle. A cycle characterised by busy-ness, anxiety and frustration with the dating app, which ultimately led to their deletion – but soon enough, their re-download. Michael's relationship was no less jagged, he discovered that stuck in this COVID-limbo, he still experienced the relationship and milestone limbo. His relationship not only lacked the milestones, but also the visibility needed for it to survive in those opening stages. There were no bars or restaurant dates, there was no meeting of the family and friends. It was almost as though the relationship could only exist within the COVID-confines.

Michael's own experience on Bumble and Tinder described the casual racism that Leo spoke too. I use the word 'casual' with intent, because participants and Michael often described it, as though it were a common-place experience, something that was expected on a dating app, nothing to be surprised about. The labour around crafting a profile that expressed the stereotype of the 'Aussie Bloke' and whiteness was again here described until Michael took to an 'Asian' specific dating app. Dating apps are often unsafe places for people that are not white, or LGBTIQ, particularly at intersectional points for example Indigenous women, and Asian queer men. However, this is rarely portrayed by contemporary media, which chooses to instead focus on patriarchal discussions around white women's safety-limiting agency.

The second anecdote describes the insidious language of PR and marketing and how it found it's way into intimacy and relationships. Celebrities started the trend of soft and hard launching relationships, however, it's now become commonplace for ordinary people to do exactly the same. And while it wasn't dating app specific, this phenomenon described some of the key findings. Finding a significant other, or being in a relationship was fundamental for the majority of the participants, some of which described how their lives had not fundamentally started because they hadn't reached this critical milestone. The soft or hard launch signifies that you've met this milestone and that you're now worthy of being someone. The significant influx of followers to Kourtney Kardashian's account exemplifies this. Once described as the 'least interesting to look at' within the Kardashian clan, her relationship with rocker Travis Barker seemed to catapult her into the world of 'interesting', and her highly documented love affair (via Instagram) was critical to this success. This documenting highlighted key relationship stages, described also in the research. They are a way of narrating a love story, or ultimately, narrativising a life. Again, this concept also described the unholy union of PR, the marketplace, labour and intimacy, so often remarked upon, again casually, within this research.

Finally, the conversation in the Uber saw the reinforcement of concepts that had emerged within the space of gender, gender scripts and stereotypes. Ideas relating to women describing themselves as brands and through consumer products were here echoed, as well as this concept of the 'high-maintenance' woman – however, this was spun in a diverse way to how I had interpreted it. In interpreting the data, it appeared that women sought to describe themselves through behavioural characteristics as opposed to appearance (which was more the domain of men). Indeed, in this case, the 'high-maintenance' component described a type of woman who was looking to have her lifestyle paid by a man, or as the Uber driver described it – a gold digger – which, notably remains a behavioural characteristic. The need for women to be pretty but low maintenance was again here validated – an impossible line that women skirted. Within this context, it was hard not to see it as, women needed to be pretty, but amenable, easy to get a long with, not demanding of too many things. It reminded me of a quote from the book *Gone Girl*, and the description of a cool girl:

> Being the Cool Girl means I am a hot, brilliant, funny woman who adores football, poker, dirty jokes, and burping, who plays video games, drinks cheap beer, loves threesomes and anal sex, and jams hot dogs and hamburgers into her mouth like she's hosting the world's biggest culinary gang bang while somehow maintaining a size 2, because Cool Girls are above all hot.

This 'high-maintenance' component didn't just translate into a focus on appearance, it meant that women needed to make themselves small to appease men on dating apps. They needed to take up as little space as possible. This congealed, sticky and gross title, meant that women were made to feel that they couldn't ask for their needs to be met, couldn't voice an opinion or appear to be difficult. They had to plaster a smile on their face, be pretty and of course low maintenance. The title was as insidious as it was demeaning in its infantilisation – that is, girls not women.

A summary of the research

Dating apps have become instrumental in how people navigate or commence intimacies. This includes hook-ups, relationships, dating and even simply, connections. As statistics described in the opening chapters of this thesis indicate, most Australians have used a dating app to navigate or facilitate an intimacy, the largest portion of these users are within the 18–35-year-old age group, which was the rationale around narrowing my sample to this age-group.

I commenced this research by conducting an auto-ethnographic baseline exercise. I call it a 'baseline' exercise – because it wasn't a deep immersion and doesn't do justice to the term auto-ethnographic. However, I have never used a dating app, and as Albury et al. (2020) a key issue for researchers and journalists documenting dating app use is a lack of familiarity with app infrastructure, and also the overall experience. Whilst Albury et al. (2020) do not make the leap to indicate that this might result in the general moral panic demonstrated by the media, however, it is safe to say this lack of first-person understanding of the apps could lead to misinterpretation and misrepresentation. As an example, dating apps are often entangled in a discourse regarding men sending dick pics, and the facilitation of such imagery via app infrastructure, when in reality, apps like Tinder do not have image-sharing capabilities. Participants within this sample indicated that nudes or dicks pics were either sent or requested when the discussion had shifted to WhatsApp or SnapChat.

To avoid this pitfall, I set up a profile on both Bumble and Tinder. I was conscious that this was also misleading as I had no intent of using the apps for their purpose. As a result, I set up a basic profile with three photos, no bio, my age and a one-word description of my profession, 'writer'. I didn't swipe on profiles, and later, bought the premium packages on both apps, as I discovered that the user had to interact with the app to gather an understanding of swiping capabilities/matching, etc. The experience gave me an understanding of how profiles were set up, what men's profiles looked like, behaviours on app, etc., and assisted in shaping the development of my questions for the focus groups.

The in-field component of my research commenced in March 2020, at the same time as Australia was plunged into the first COVID-19 lockdown. My aim was to conduct two iterative semi-structure focus groups to gather an understanding of how the groups perceived dating apps, intimacy and the construction of gender on dating apps, as well as thing out any new or different ideas relating to dating apps that hadn't been accounted for in my research development. These two groups were conducted face-to-face; however, the spectre of COVID and a COVID lockdown was already looming, as well as the idea of loneliness, compressed milestones and even the need to find an iso-partner.

Participants were asked set questions in the first focus group around their dating app experience, usage practices, personal presentation on apps, expectations and desires. Questions were tailored for the second focus group around trends that emerged, and participants were also asked to design their ideal dating app architecture and functionalities in groups.

Sixteen in-depth interviews were then conducted over Zoom and were approximately an hour in length, following a semi-structured format. Eight participants also journaled their experience during the month of March and were asked to do so for at least one hour per week, capturing screen grabs of their experience if they desired.

Twenty participants were recruited: twelve were heterosexual women, six were heterosexual men and two were queer men. Two participants were consensually non-monogamous, the rest were 'single' or were in the preliminary stages of dating ('talking to') someone. The research intended on capturing heterosexual dating app practices, although it did not seek to exclude other sexualities or ways of being.

To gather an understanding of the prevalent media narratives which were being narrated at the time of data collection, a media audit across March and April 2020 (broadcast, digital and print), using iSentia. Keywords were established such as Bumble, Tinder, dating, dating apps, intimacy and relationships. The aim was to monitor the contemporary media narrative and overlay this with data from the focus groups, interviews and e-journals to see intersections in themes, keywords and narratives.

Overall key findings and their complexities

COVID-19: the compression of time accordion style and love milestones

COVID-19 was a difficult external player to ignore in the shaping of users' experience on dating apps during 2020. As indicated, I began my research in March

2020, and at the same time, we were plunged into the first COVID lockdown – my focus groups conducted in person, the rest of the research via zoom.

It quickly became clear that dating apps were going to play a key role during COVID-19. In mid-March, the Australian media were captured by major apps Public Service Announcements re-COVID. Most apps delivered an in-app PSA about COVID, directing their audience towards the WHO guidelines on how to keep COVID safe. Whilst initially this was a source of humour, the laughter was quickly silenced. Dating apps recorded extreme increases in usage, and users similarly corroborated this activity. One participant said, her phone was 'pinging off the hook' as a result of new matches, and another noted, that he had not seen a new face on a dating app (as he had limited search results to a 10km radius), but now '... there are all these new faces'. This reflected that there was more activity on dating apps, and also, more new sign-ups.

Many studies have been developed to identify how confinement has impacted the health of the world population, aiming at identifying possible relationships between psychosocial, psychological and behavioural changes during the confinement period and obtaining scientific data that could help to characterise the psychosocial aspects of the COVID-19 crisis. In general, the authors describe how the COVID-19 pandemic has impacted the mental health of citizens worldwide; isolation measures, fear, uncertainty, and economic turmoil, lack of social connectedness and trust in other people and institutions, and jobs and incomes being at risk are taking a huge toll in terms of anxiety and worry, leading to 'psychological distress'. The United Nations (UN) has warned of the necessity for a policy briefing, calling for substantial investment in support services. Depression and anxiety cost the global economy more than one trillion dollars per year, and this was before the COVID-19 pandemic, and globally the ratio of mental health professionals per citizen is 1 to 10,000 (Clemente-Suárez et al., 2020). It was impossible not to frame the research findings against and through the lens of the COVID-19 pandemic, as the data were collected during the first lockdown in NSW, and there was a clear interplay or correlation between the findings and the pragmatic and psychosocial impacts of the pandemic.

COVID-19 in this case appeared to have multiple affects on participants, the first was pragmatic, they could no longer meet people face-to-face, and this made dating apps one of the few places available to them to meet a significant other, which drove the uptake of dating apps, as well as the increased activity.

However, alongside this, for many of the participants within this sample, there was a heightened awareness of their singleness during the COVID-19 lockdown and a sense that they had not met critical life milestones. For example, one participant indicated she had a sense that her 'life hadn't really started' because she hadn't been involved in a significant relationship or 'settled down'. This participant equated the critical milestone of meeting a significant other, alongside finding the right job, both of these elements had to occur for her to have a sense of life commencing. COVID-19 appeared to exacerbate this sense of life-inertia. Working from homes, participants lives were no longer punctuated by dinners, movies and parties, the busy-ness that Bauman identifies as part of the 'liquid modern' was removed from their everyday lives. As a result, there was a sense of stagnancy, or as many participants mentioned 'wasting time'. This temporal anxiety indicated that participants believed there was a 'good way' and a 'bad way' to spend time, and the good way was characterised by meeting life milestones – during the COVID-19 lockdown this achievement of life goals was removed. As a result, participants replaced the busy-ness of Bauman's liquid modern, with the busy-ness of dating app usage. Downloading, swiping, DM'ing consistently, seemingly with no outcomes.

The participant who said her phone was 'pinging off the hook' with messages from potential matches, however, she also indicated that using dating apps was 'exhausting', and likened her apps to 'going back to work to find your inbox full'. This (what can only be described as dread) of trailing through hundreds of messages banked up in the Direct Message chat was common to participants. Taj similarly described the 'anxiety of seeing the three little dots … you know they're writing something and you have to respond'. This went towards the labour of using dating apps during COVID-19.

For participants, there was a sense that everyone single was currently on dating apps, and this was the only way to meet someone at this point in time. Hence, they needed to be on a dating app. They needed to be participating in the noise of the dating app environment, and in addition they had to dial up their usage. However, they experienced stress, anxiety and even dread when it came to interacting with the dating app. The labour of yet another digital experience – alongside the work from home zoom fatigue, the updating of Instagram, Facebook and even TikTok – was extreme and overwhelming. For many it ended in tears.

There was a tension here for participants. Many used dating apps to alleviate boredom during the COVID-19 lockdown, hence they were also a source of distraction, levity and even joy. They described it as a quick and easy way to interact with someone, experience the frivolity and fun of a short flirtation, or even simply of a connection. However, these experiences were juxtaposed to heavier ones, for example, never-ending messaging chats, filled with a mundanity and minutiae. In this case, dating apps were more like, as one participant described, 'a second job'.

The COVID-19 lockdown appeared to amplify both of these tensions. The time away from work and even simple interactions that participants usually would have had at the coffee shop, for example, meant that their connections were limited. The interactions with other human beings, even via a dating app, were sorely needed and appreciated. At the same time, the urge to participate in this maelstrom of dating app activity and to achieve an outcome – that is, a feasible match, meant they often over-swiped, over-DM'd and generally, over-participated, which enhanced the sense that they were working, that dating apps were a second job, that the labour of dating apps was too much to deal with, which all went towards the jagged love cycle, and *the love/hate relationship with the dating apps* as opposed to with another human being.

Romantic Narrative in the dating app space

A surprising finding within this research was the persistence of romantic masterplot(s) within participants understanding of how a relationship should unfold, and also in relation to how participants used dating apps. Notably, the idea of the romantic masterplot(s) has consistently come under challenge across the last three decades, particularly through post-feminist reads of romantic fiction, for example by McRobbie (1997), Smith (2011) and Johnson (1997) – all of which grappled with the idea of women becoming women through consumption (often detailed through romantic fiction) as opposed to traditional romantic masterplot(s). As Johnson indicates (1997) in relation to a study of a series of novels ascribed to the romantic-fiction category:

> The central finding of this study is that these teen and tween romance novels created by Alloy have departed from the genre's former narrative focus. Reflecting the marketing focus of Alloy Media Marketing "total immersion" of brands in everyday life and similar to magazine "advertorials," consumption of branded goods and services in these entertaining narratives is directly linked to obtaining romantic relationships. While romance still remains an important aspect of the heroines' lives, the overriding focus is the process of continuous consumption, mostly of expensive products and services, to strive for romantic success and competitive edge against other girls. Heroines no longer, as Christian-Smith (1988, 1990) asserted, become women through romance, they now become empowered and feminine through consumption.

McRobbie built on these ideas of women being empowered and defined through consumption, by also describing a right-way to leave, through life goals and achievements, for example getting an education, the ideal job, consuming the right products, and also having the right relationship. Threads of these ideas were persistent through the research, women defined themselves more so through behavioural characteristics on app, then through appearance (for example being a young professional, or sporty), however, they also often meshed together romantic milestones, with perceived neo-liberalist milestones, like finding the right job.

However, the persistence of romantic masterplot(s) narrative and milestones, both for women and men within this sample, was evident. One of the key elements which was consistently raised was the need for some sort of 'meet cute' to herald the start of an important relationship. Participants would often reference rom-coms in relation to how they understood the 'meet cute' to work, a happenstance coming together of an unlikely duo, always notably, in a face-to-face environment. Many also indicated that their friends and family members had met their significant other in a pseudo meet-cute and as a result they felt they were falling short of these lofty love ideals, by meeting someone via a dating app. The dating app environment conflicted with how an important relationship should start because there was nothing happenstance or unexpected about the dating app environment, it was pre-meditated and strategic. Many participants had the sense that they weren't good-looking enough, funny, or intelligent enough to have a meet-cute. For example, Yasmin indicate, 'I'm not the type of person who starts talking to someone at the cafe or on the bus … I don't think I'm good looking enough and I'm kind of an awkward person'. There was a sense that meet-cutes and the romantic narrative were open to people who were more capable, generally at life. Despite the knowledge that most people were on dating apps, the majority of participants had the sense that they had failed from a romantic perspective, and this was evident through their dating app usage. This again was amplified by COVID. Participants had a sense that key milestones should have been met by now, particularly during the inertia of COVID-19, and finding a love interest was one of them, now, and as a result of COVID-19 they might be destined to be alone. Alex said, 'Do I get the sense that the clock is ticking? Yes, absolutely. And now, its worse, because of COVID, everything has come to a halt'.

This temporal anxiety, the sense that life milestones should happen at a particular time, and in an order, was expressed by many participants. The sense that COVID-19 was playing havoc with this intended pathway, also indicated. One participant said, 'I feel like now I'm about to miss another year from a love year … another year where I haven't met someone'.

Here, the participant indicated a projected romantic time frame that had to be met – straight time. However, the uncertainty of how long we could be in a lockdown was another point of contention for participants in the negotiation of intimacy online. Another element to the dating app is melange, which will later be described.

Participants were even annoyed they had to use a dating app. One participant summarised this well,

> I don't find dating apps empowering. I have the shits that I have to use them. Like, I have no other options. Nobody meets face to face anymore, and nobody introduces anyone anymore. So where else am I going to meet someone?

There was a frustration for Roxanne, she didn't want to participate in the dating app loop, but she had to.

Shumway described how we narrativise life as a series of stories, with key events and milestones. Whilst these events and milestones have consistently been challenged, it is notable that participants reflected the love narrative was critical to their life progression. To some degree, this is seen through the success of the romantic narrative on Instagram. Kourtney Kardashian gained over 40 million followers after she announced her new relationship, and mobilised the correct cultural codifiers to do so. The romantic narrative continues to have cultural primacy and right and wrong ways for it to be expressed. This isn't to say that the narrative isn't under challenge, or that diverse narratives don't exist, however, within this research it was indelible. I could hypothesise that this was because of COVID-19, that the uncertainty of the period, made participants cling to known romantic narratives, however, I don't have evidence to this effect. Notably, the consensually non-monogamous couple within this sample shifted to being monogamous during COVID-19, which could indicate a need to return to known relationship paradigms, however, this change was likely also pragmatic.

Another persistent trope, which was raised by participants, was that one shouldn't have to look for love. Again, this fell into a narrative around love being happenstance, magic almost, irreducible to a set of algorithms and formulas. As a result the consistent labour that participants had to deploy to use dating apps – conflicted with this masterplot and created a tension of sorts for them. They were aware that dating apps were the only place for them to meet someone at this point in time, but they were quite sure that dating apps couldn't deliver against the romantic narrative that they sort. As a result, they occupied a strange but familiar post-modernist space, they were occupied in labour (in this case of finding love), but they were quite aware that this labour could not yield the result they were after. They were just working, but feared leaving the dating app paradigm, because there were simply no other options.

Bauman and Jagged Love

Bauman's ideas on Liquid Love and the Liquid Modern were important to the development of this work. First, because there were so many similarities in his description of Liquid Love and the findings within this research, but also because of the tensions and points of difference.

For Bauman, modernity has ushered in a new paradigm for lovers, where people consume partners or intimacy, like they would consume clothes or food. Quickly becoming intrigued by them, and intimate and almost at the speed, moving on and discarding of the person – and so, onto the next. Dating apps or computer-mediated dating is symptomatic of this unique condition, as users are able to rotate through a virtual market of individuals, sampling and discarding at whim. Bauman described a particular type of anxiety that is caused by this behaviour. First, love and intimacy continues to be seen as the pinnacle of life and achievement in contemporary culture. Hence the quest for a committed relationship is still the primary indicator of a 'good life', or in a narritivised version, a 'happily ever after'. The yearning for the stability of a relationship, is juxtaposed against this veritable buffet of individuals, of desire, and of course, of lack of commitment. Bauman draws on Kundera and his ideas around the tension of lightness/lack of burden versus heaviness and shackles. To lead a good life is to set up foundations, to leave something significant behind, but this tethering is at tension with the liquid modern, with consumption, joy and freedom. Bauman describes how people shift through this liquid modern paradigm, smoothly, easily, shifting from partner to partner, in a never-ending sample of affairs and people.

Essential to Bauman's theory is the idea of busy-ness. The notion that we come to be owned by the busy-ness without the outcome. The endless lunch dates, dinners, emails, phone calls and life admin. We participate in the busy-ness, simply to be part of the busy-ness, and to no longer participate, is to be annihilated as an individual, to no longer be relevant.

Many of Bauman's theoretical musings were present in this research. For example, participants did come to be defined by the busy-ness of the dating apps. They felt they needed to participate (otherwise they would never find a match, a prerequisite to a worthy life), but in contrast, they also were burdened by the non-stop messaging, the constant labour that was required to participate. As previously indicated they came to be categorised by that labour and busy-ness, rather than by the experience. But, of course, there was complexity here, because the dating apps also brought them on occasion joy and connection.

The majority of participants in this same participated in the liquid modern, but had firm views on love and life (as indicated in the persistence of the romantic narrative). They believed in the need to find a significant other. In Kundera and Bauman's solidity, in fact they were anxious to find this, anxious to get away from the rotating door that was dating apps, but frustrated that they had been shoe-horned into a space where they had to participate in the dating app paradigm. There was nothing liquid about their transition from one fling or match to the next. The process was harrowing. There were tears and anger, and many would break-up with the dating apps themselves as a result.

For participants, the dating apps came to embody their source of frustration. Their stymied efforts of finding love, the COVID-19 inertia, the lack of intimacy – for participants, this was a result of the dating apps. As one participant described, they forged a 'love/hate relationship with the dating apps' – and what I came to term, the jagged love cycle. They would download multiple apps, upload profiles, swipe 'savagely', DM to the point of exhaustion, but nothing would ever eventuate. Long-term intimacy was illusive on the dating apps, and as a result participants would often take a break from the apps, deleting all of them, almost spitefully from their phones. To some degree, it was almost as though the apps were animate, and this action was taken to hurt them. Eventually, usually after a couple of weeks participants would experience a sense of FOMO and re-download the apps – the cycle commencing all over again.

It was jagged in nature. One participant said, 'I've never cried this much in my life'. Another said, 'The apps give me the shits'. And finally, one said, 'I used to think I was an ok looking bloke until I got on the dating apps. Now I feel pretty shit about myself'. There was no fluidity, no seamless progression from one conversation or match to the next, it was staccato in nature, angry and also sad. Again, this can be problematised because the dating apps did provide participants a sense of entertainment and connectivity during COVID-19.

In summation: they were loved and hated, all at the same time.

Negotiating intimacy online

The negotiation of intimacy in the online environment was problematic for the majority of participants. For Berlant and Giddens, intimacy involves a mutual sharing, whether it be a sharing of secrets, affects, or potential life trajectories. Intimacy involves the sharing of something deep within us, which isn't usually shared with others. One participant expressed this darkly, when asked what intimacy was he indicated that it was showing the other person how 'fucked up you really are'. To this participant, intimacy was almost akin to Goffman's idea of the frontstage and backstage, the backstage being the stage occupied when being intimacy. During the focus groups I asked all participants what intimacy meant to them, and most referred to sharing (secrets in particular), or being able to be yourself, a capacity to be vulnerable, or being the person behind the veneer. While Jakub's expression of intimacy was a crude one, it seemed to summarise the overall sentiments. I then asked participants if they thought finding an intimacy was possible on a dating app, or developing an intimacy – the majority said no. The responses were similar, no, and then a rue smile, as though they all had a shared understanding of the dating app experience. That said, a few in the sample indicated otherwise.

Ultimately, participants felt that the dating app landscape was a shallow one, that didn't allow for the development of an intimacy. Decisions were made quickly, usually based on appearance, or other cultural codifiers expressed via the profile. Participants also indicated that they were more judgmental in the dating app landscape, far more than they would be IRL. Bek indicated that while she made quick decisions on matches, 'Next, next, next …' IRL she would consider a person in a deeper way. Participants thought this was largely due to the app infrastructure – the plethora of people, described largely only, by a series of images. However, later in in-depth interviews it became clearer that it was a combination of both the infrastructure, as well as how participants used datings apps.

The majority of people sought an intimate relationship via dating apps, with the exception of the consensually non-monogamous couple, and some participants who had hook-up profiles, alongside relationship profiles. There was a general sense that a hook-up couldn't develop into a relationship – for this reason, the two profiles were kept separate by the majority of participants (withstanding queer men). This could have been because relationship milestones were shuffled (if the hook-up occurred first) or simply because the hook-up details had to be negotiated assiduously, and pertained to only the one interaction. With hook-ups participants indicated they were clear, direct, about when, how and what, however, with relationships or a deeper intimacy, this communication became nebulous. The majority of participants identified several critical impediments for developing an intimacy: the first was that they invested at a low level with multiple people. This meant that conversations were often mundane, and categorised by minutiae, the type of discussion that was 'How has your day been?' As opposed to the deeper stuff that might have facilitated sharing, but also been exciting enough, and in line with participants romantic narrative. This lack of investment was a form of self-preservation (not putting all your eggs in one basked) or as Stuart indicated, 'keeping your numbers high, to avoid obsessing over the one person'. However, it was counter-intuitive, it resulted in more labour of participants – the consistent responding to of irrelevant messages.

Participants also described a certain lack of what I came to describe as 'animation'. An ineffable sort of quality – where something vital to their personality, and in effect the potential chemistry with a match was lost in translation on dating app. Repeatedly the words, 'I don't translate on dating apps' were used by participants. It was almost as thought something critical to their character couldn't be communicated in the two dimensional format (a series of photos, and a bio). Many talked about how there was a lack of movement, and as a result small personality traits or quirks couldn't be converted, like how they walked, or if they talked with their hands, or even how they laughed. Movement and sound were lacking. Interestingly, most dating apps provide participants with the capacity to upload video content (Tinder and Bumble), however, participants thought this was try-hardish, and went against the grain of the romantic narrative of not trying to hard. Some referred to using platforms like TikTok to meet a match, and that more of the essential elements of a persons personality could be conveyed here. I equated the missing quality to 'animation', a term derived from the Latin term 'animare', which indeed means to be set into motion, but also means to have life aspirated into – in fact, the Latin root also equates to the soul or 'anima'. It was almost as though in lacking movement, and sound, a life-like quality was lost. The dating app space seemed to flatten people, and they simply became 'profiles', lacking the animation required to create chemistry or intimacy.

Arguably, the other reason they might have thought Instagram, TikTok, or LinkedIn were more fruitful spaces for a digital intimacy, is because the intention of these platforms is not dating or relationships – this means the initial meeting fulfils the 'happenstance' quality required in the romantic masterplot(s). The dating app *intentional* element appeared to work counter-intuitively. The requirement for elements like chemistry and an ineffable magic quality was required by participants – and the dating apps couldn't deliver this. Notably, this was not true of all participants, some of which did develop intimate connections in the dating app environment, but notably all of these ended in heartache.

It was clear that for the majority of participants there was an element of using apps out of boredom. There seemed to be a need to participate in the dating app busy-ness, even if this meant just swiping, and not interacting, or keeping up multiple surface-level discussions, which continues Bauman's theory on Liquid Love and busy-ness – that is, participants came to belong to the texts, the swiping, the participating in the dating app noise as opposed to making a lasting connection. However, notably, the incapacity to build intimacy in the dating app environment fed into the jagged love cycle, the anxiety and ultimately the hate/deletion of dating apps – only to re-upload profiles in a short period of time. COVID, again, exacerbated these tensions, as participants worried about investing in one person, without face-to-face proof that chemistry existed. In addition, the uncertainty around when the COVID lockdown might end made it further difficult for participants – would it be 6 weeks or 12 months? Here many participants reflected on the labour of dating apps – the idea they had to spend too much time managing their romantic life online, and yet conversely this labour was pitched in the wrong direction. They spread themselves thin across multiple matches, coming to belong to the busy-ness of the app as opposed to investing in the one person.

Gender stereotypes – subversions and reinforcements

That dating apps might encourage the use of heteronormative gender stereotypes was by no means a revolutionary finding. As many researchers have previously identified, dating app architecture is based on binary gender definitions, not because this is necessarily required, but because there is significant developer, company and overall biases in this space. In addition, the notion that certain apps are largely based on visual decisions, means that the environment drives a certain visual economy and a known series of cultural codifiers which could be described as hetero-sexy (both for men and women). Participants were largely attuned to this idea and were conscious in their image selection that they were seeking outcomes i.e. matches. However, there were multiple gender subversions that were of interest within this project, as well as the surfacing of notions like the 'Aussie Bloke' which were surprising.

The Aussie Bloke was a term used by both men and women, heterosexual and queer. If the term wasn't explicitly used, there were other descriptors intimated. Women and queer men indicated that the Aussie Bloke was desirable, while as heterosexual men tried to embody this notion. The idea entailed several elements. The Aussie Bloke was humorous, tall, had a beard (and other body hair) muscular, white (but tanned), he had friends or mates and he drank beer (although the latter element was challenged, men thought the Aussie Bloke drank beer, women saw this as evidence of toxic musculinity). Initially, I used Linzi Murrie's conceptualisation of the Aussie Bloke as a starting point for this identity. Steeped in corporeality, the Aussie Bloke, was strong and silent and belonged to nature and not culture. Indeed, the Aussie Bloke has been used across the centuries, he has been the Larrikin, the Anzac and also John Howard's working-class hero.

Australian historian Russel Ward in *The Australian Legend* (1958) described the mythical 'Aussie bloke' as:

> ...a practical man, rough and ready in his manners and quick to decry any appearance of affectation in others... Though capable of great exertion in an emergency, he normally feels no impulse to work hard without good cause. He swears hard and consistently, gambles heavily and often, and drinks deeply on occasion... he is a greater knocker of eminent people unless, as is in the case of his sporting heroes, they are distinguished by

> physical prowess. He is fiercely independent… above all he will stick to his mates through thick and thin, even if he thinks they may be wrong… He tends to be a rolling stone, highly suspect if he should chance to gather much moss.

Here, the Aussie Bloke is described less through physicality and more through behavioural traits.

There seemed to be persistent character traits that were retained by the Aussie Bloke described by participants and new incorporations, like the beard and body hair, which was more a reflection of the modern day city slicker or hipster (which ran counter to the narrative of the Aussie Bloke belonging to nature rather than culture). There were tensions in the definition as well, for example, the appearance of too many beers in a profile, or mates, embodied toxic masculinity for women but not for men. Similarly, there was othering, the Aussie Bloke was white and those ethnically diverse felt they could never really embody the characteristics. As Leo indicated, 'I can't change that I'm Asian'.

The Aussie Bloke was as slippery as it was othering. None of the men in the research felt like they did justice to the character, and as a result constantly had the sense that they were doing masculinity incorrectly. However, their focus was on the visual. They didn't shy away from indicating they were hyper-focussed on their visual identity or using tools like filters and FaceTune to achieve these outcomes – which tended to subvert ideas of men being grounded in doing as opposed to the physical. There was also an elevated vulnerability in men around their dating app profiles. Men indicated they felt 'shit' about themselves generally when they interacted with dating apps and had a strong sense they were performing masculinity incorrectly. They didn't use other men as benchmarks for their profiles, instead, they relied on the number of matches they received, which tended to indicate their profiles were guided by the female lens.

Contrarily, women based their profiles on behavioural traits, looking to portray themselves as professional, sporty, or even musos. The important part as one participant indicated was that she was a girl that 'did stuff' and this was conveyed through her profile. To some degree, this sat aligned with McRobbie's idea of the post-feminist woman, grounded in consumption, but also in white, middle-class milestones, like getting an education, and the right job. However, there was something energetic about women's profiles, and even, empowered. They were less focussed on appearances and more on what constituted themselves as a person. Women often described themselves as a brand. As Bek indicated re nudes, 'that's off brand for me', which fell into McRobbie's consumption narrative, but also into a broader dialogue around dating apps, which encourage users to market themselves as brands, mobilising key cultural codifiers.

Women were less concerned by the male lens and instead were focussed on the female. They often used friends, sibling,s or even their mothers to check their profiles. For many, this fell into a culture of care exercise, where female friends would have dinner and discuss their profiles, and have a laugh. Yasmin indicated that she asked her friends to write her bio. She believed this to be the most intimate part of her profile and thought her friends knew her almost better than herself. For one participant, this female lens served to reinforce concepts around hyper femininity – that is, her mother indicated that she needed to dial up more feminine cultural codifiers (like wearing a dress). This caused conflict for this participant, who had always struggled with defining herself as a woman, and had always been described as, 'tom-boyish'.

The majority of participants (and men more so than women) felt that they were performing a particular attractive interpretation of themselves in the dating app environment, and this led to anxieties and vulnerabilities. These were perhaps more keenly felt within the COVID vacuum, which made us also consider our lives in more detail, and what we should have, or would have wanted to achieve by 2020. For the majority of participants, this was having a significant relationship.

Overall, there was a sense of anxiety and vulnerability in portraying self on the apps. There was a labour involved here. A consistent monitoring and curating profiles to ensure they struck the right note, which meant that labour, romance and intimacy became heavily intertwined.

Dating apps as spaces to find intimacy and everything else

I began this project with the aim to learn whether dating apps change the way intimacies are navigated and negotiated. Explicitly, I was looking to gather an understanding of how and if dating apps reinforced or subverted gender stereotypes. Like most researchers, I entered this arena with own pre-conceived stereotypes, that I dared not mention to other, but were notwithstanding, buried deep within me. After all, I too had consumed the media hysteria around dating apps, the moral panic around how dating apps were cheapening love, making it a meat market, and of course, that they were dangerous places, particularly for women. I'd also heard my fair share of stories about creepy guys, and of course, the notorious dick pics.

What I came to learn with dating apps was indeed something quite different. As Condie indicates, dating apps are, 'Messy and muddled, complex and consuming, Tinder is completely inseparable from the people who use it'.

Never was this more obvious than in COVID times, when participants relied on dating apps for the majority of connections but also felt temporal anxieties around missed milestones – never having met the one, never having really started life. Stuck in the COVID inertia – they looked to regain a sense of momentum, and dating apps provided an avenue. They were a road to meet a significant other and to kick-start the romantic narrative, they were a way to re-engage in the busy-ness of life as they knew it, and they were also a way to create sorely needed connections.

But for most dating apps didn't provide the narrative they sought. The architecture itself was at odds with the romantic narrative they expected. The strategy butted against the happenstance needs of love – love after all happens when you're not looking for it. They were surfaced key issues, vulnerabilities and anxieties, lack of worth (particularly for men), a need to perform certain concepts of masculinity and brand behavioural traits, which were difficult, slippery, impossible even, to embody. And this furthered the angst.

Instead of fluidly moving in a love, sex and intimacy conveyer belt, Bauman-style, they found themselves in violent, staccato shifts, experiencing joy, sadness, anger, hate, glimpses of intimacy and all the rest, one and at the same time. Setting into motion what I came to term, the jagged love cycle, a loop, a love/hate relationship with the apps, where the apps came to embody everything that they hated and loved about themselves.

Conversely to what was anticipated, dating apps did not turn out to be an unsafe place for white women (as often portrayed in the media), but they were equally unsafe for others within this sample. Surfaced within this research was the casual racism expressed on dating apps, the idea that Bumble and Tinder are apps explicitly intended for white people.

Dating apps are presented as a melange of things. A place to connect, perform, interact, be busy, experience joy and anger, and for some find love and intimacy. They were not one thing, but many.

A catch-all of sorts for the digital experience.

Overall: messy.

REFERENCES

7News. (2020). "Sydney Man Faces Court over Alleged Rape of Tinder Date." https://7news.com.au/news/nsw/sydney-man-faces-court-over-alleged-rape-of-tinder-date-c-1436274

Aapola, Sinikka, Marnina Gonick, and Anita Harris. (2005). *Young Femininity: Girlhood, Power, and Social Change.* New York: Palgrave.

Abbott, H. Porter. (2008). *The Cambridge Introduction to Narrative.* Cambridge: Cambridge University Press.

ABC. (2020, 8 October). *Tinder: How Digital Dating became a Predators Playground.* https://www.abc.net.au/news/2020-10-08/tinder:-how-digital-dating-became-a-predators%E2%80%99/12744980?nw=0

Abdin, Crystal. (2014). "#In$tagLam: Instagram as a Repository of Taste, a Burgeoning Marketplace, a War of Eyeballs." In *Mobile Media Making in an Age of Smartphones,* edited by M. Berry and M. Schleser, 119–128. New York: Palgrave.

Adkins, Lisa, and Celia Lury. (2011). "Introduction: Special Measures." *The Sociological Review* 59 (2, Suppl.): 5–23. SAGE Journals.

AFP. (2019, June 8). "Dating Apps and STDs: A Million New Sexually Transmitted Infections a Day, WHO Warns." https://www.scmp.com/lifestyle/health-wellness/article/3013588/dating-apps-and-stds-million-new-sexually-transmitted

Albright, Julie M., and Steve Carter. (2019). "The Myth of the Siren's Song: Gendered Courtship and Sexual Scripts in Online Dating." In *It Happened on Tinder: Reflections and Studies on Internet-Infused Dating,* edited by Amir Hetsroni and Meriç Tuncez, 10–30. Amsterdam: INC.

Albury, Kath. (2019). "Dating Apps are the Norm and Its Time to Stop Viewing Them as a Risk." https://www.swinburne.edu.au/news/2019/12/dating-apps-are-the-norm-and-its-time-to-stop-viewing-them-as-a-risk/

Albury, Kath, et al. (2019). "Safety, Risk and Wellbeing on Dating Apps: Final Report." Output from the Australian Research Council Linkage Project 'Safety, Risk and Wellbeing on Digital Dating Apps,' published first online, DOI: 10.25916/5dd324c1b33bb.

Albury, Kath, Anthony McCosker, Tinonee Pym, and Paul Byron. (2020). "Dating Apps as Public Health 'problems': Cautionary Tales and Vernacular Pedagogies in New Media." *Health Sociology Review* 29 (3): 232–248. DOI: 10.1080/14461242.2020.1777885.

Albury, Kath, Jean Burgess, Ben Light, Kane Race, and Rowan Wilken. (2017). "Data Cultures of Mobile Dating and Hook-up Apps: Emerging Issues for Critical Social Science Research." *Big Data & Society* 4 (2), published first online. DOI: 10.1177/2053951717720950.

Albury, Kath, and Kate Crawford. (2012). "Sexting, Consent and Young People's Ethics: Beyond Megan's Story." Taylor and Francis Online. DOI: 10.1080/10304312.2012.665840

Altheide, David L., and John M. Johnson. (1994). "Criteria for Assessing Interpretive Validity in Qualitative Research." In *Handbook of Qualitative Research*, edited by Norman K. Denzin and Yvonna S. Lincoln, 485–499. Washington, DC: Sage Publications, Inc.

Amanpour, Christiane. (2020). *Sex and Love around the World*, Netflix series.

Ammar, Achraf, et al. (2020). "Psychological Consequences of COVID-19 Home Confinement: The ECLB-COVID19 Multicenter Study." *PLoS ONE* 15 (11): e0240204.

Austen, Jane. (1811). *Sense and Sensibility*. Thomas Egerton: Military Library (Whitehall, London).

Austen, Jane. (1815). *Emma*. Thomas Egerton: Military Library (Whitehall, London).

Australian Institute of Health and Welfare. (2020). "Sexual Assault in Australia." https://www.aihw.gov.au/getmedia/0375553f-0395-46cc-9574-d54c74fa601a/aihw-fdv-5.pdf.aspx?inline=true

Avery, Jessica. (2018, December 27). *A Beginner's Guide to Forced Proximity Romance Novels*. Book Riot. https://bookriot.com/forced-proximity-romance-novels/

Ayers, C. (2014). "Tinder: The App that is Setting the Dating Scene on Fire." Accessed 29 February 2015. http://www.theaustralian.com.au/life/weekend-australian-magazine/tinder-the-app-thatssetting-the-dating-scene-on-fire/story-e6frg8h6-1226933263450

Bacchi, Carol. (2016). "Problematizations in Health Policy: Questioning How "Problems" Are Constituted in Policies." First Published June 1, 2016 Research Article. DOI: 10.1177/2158244016653986

Badal, Hannah J., Jo E. Stryker, Nickolas DeLuca, et al. (2018). "Swipe Right: Dating Website and App Use among Men Who Have Sex with Men." *AIDS and Behavior* 22: 1265–1272. DOI: 10.1007/s10461-017-1882-7

Bailey, John. (2012). "Changing the Game." *The Age*, February 12. Accessed 19 July 2021. https://www.theage.com.au/lifestyle/changing-the-game-20120211-1sy90.html#ixzz1mTfkGD2D

Banet-Weiser, Sarah. (2012). *Authentic TM: The Politics and Ambivalence in a Brand Culture*. New York: New York University Press.

Banet-Weiser, Sarah. (2018). *Empowered: Popular Feminism and Popular Misogyny*. Durham, NC: Duke University Press.

Barad, Karen. (2003). "Posthumanist Performativity. Toward an Understanding of How Matter Comes to Matter." *Signs* 28: 801–831.

Barad, Karen. (2007). *Meeting the Universe Halfway*. Durham, NC: Duke University Press.

Bartky, Sandra L. (1988). *Femininity and Domination: Studies in the Phenomenology of Oppression*. New York: Routledge.

Bauman, Zygmunt. (2003). *Liquid Love: On the Frailty of Human Bonds*. Cambridge: Polity.

BBC. (2021, March). "Australian March 4 Justice: Thousands March against Sexual Assault." https://www.bbc.com/news/world-australia-56397170

BBC. (2021, March). "How Rape Allegations Have Rocked Australian Politics." https://www.bbc.com/news/world-australia-56178290

Benjamin, Walter. (1935). *The Work of Art in the Age of Mechanical Reproduction*. Brodersen XV, London: Penguin.

Bennett, Jane. (2009). *Vibrant Matter: A Political Ecology of Things*. Durham, NC: Duke University Press.

Benotsch, Eric G., Daniel J. Snipes, Aaron M. Martin, and Sheana S. Bull. (2013 March). "Sexting, Substance Use, and Sexual Risk Behavior in Young Adults." *Journal of Adolescent Health* 52 (3): 307–313. DOI: 10.1016/j.jadohealth.2012.06.011. Epub 2012 August 14. PMID: 23299017; PMCID: PMC3580005.

Belsey, Catherine. (1994). *Desire: Love Stories in Western Culture*. Oxford: Wiley Blackwell.

Berlant, Lauren. (1998). "Intimacy: A Special Issue." *Critical Inquiry* 24 (2): 281–288. DOI: 10.1086/448875.

Bertoni, Steven. (2014). "Tinder Swipes Right to Revenue, Will Add Premium Service in November, Forbes." https://www.forbes.com/sites/stevenbertoni/2014/10/20/tinder-swipes-right-to-revenue-will-add-premium-service-in-november/?sh=7832128e1ee0

Best, Shaun. (2019). "Liquid Love: Zygmunt Bauman's Thesis on Sex Revisited." *Sexualities* 22 (7–8): 1094–1109. DOI: 10.1177/1363460718795082.

Bivens, Rena, and Anna S. Hoque. (2018). "Programming Sex, Gender, and Sexuality: Infrastructural Failures in the 'feminist' Dating App Bumble." *Canadian Journal of Communication* 43 (3): 441–459. DOI: 10.22230/cjc.2019v44n3a3375

Blackwell, Courtney. (2014). "Seeing and Being Seen: Co-situation and Impression Formation Using Grindr, a Location-Aware Gay Dating App." *News and Media and Society*. DOI: 10.1177/1461444814521595

Boellstorff, Tom. (2007). "When Marriage Falls." *GLQ: A Journal of Lesbian & Gay Studies* 13 (2–3): 227–248. DOI: 10.1215/10642684-2006-032.

Bogle, Kathleen A. (2008). *Hooking up: Sex, Dating, and Relationships on Campus*. New York: New York University Press.

Bonos, Lisa. (2018). "Why Are Tinder and Bumble Fighting? Here's Everything You Need to Know." https://www.washingtonpost.com/news/soloish/wp/2018/03/22/why-are-tinder-and-bumble-fighting-its-been-a-long-and-winding-feud/

Bowers, Jack. (2017). "Lest We Forget: Mateship, Masculinity and Australian Identity." In *Mediating Memory: Tracing the Limits of Memoir*, edited by Bunty Avieson, Fiona Giles, and Sue Joseph, 299–314. Abingdon: Routledge. DOI: 10.4324/9781315107349.

Boyd, Danah. (2009). "The Not-So-Hidden Politics of Class Online." (Personal Blog) https://www.danah.org/papers/talks/PDF2009.html

Boydell, Katherine. (2010). *A descriptive review of qualitative studies in first episode psychosis*. Wiley Online Library.

Braidotti, Rosi. (2018). "A Theoretical Framework for the Critical Posthumanities." *Theory, Culture & Society*. Advance online publication. DOI: 10.1177/0263276418771486

Brainz. (2011). "History of Online Dating." https://www.brainz.org/history-online-dating/

Briggs, Charles L., and Daniel C. Hallin. (2010). "Health Reporting as Political Reporting: Biocommunicability and the Public Sphere." DOI: 10.1177/1464884909355732

Brisbane Times. (2020). "Brisbane Man Now Accused of Raping 21 Women He Met on Dating Apps." https://www.brisbanetimes.com.au/national/queensland/brisbane-man-now-accused-of-raping-21-women-he-met-on-dating-apps-20201209-p56m3u.html

Bronte, Emily. (1847). *Wuthering Heights*. London: Thomas Cautley Newby.

Brooks, Peter. (1996). "The Law as Narrative and Rhetoric." In *Law's Stories: Narrative and Rhetoric in the Law*, edited by Peter Brooks and Paul Gerwitz, 14–23. New Haven, CT: Yale University Press.

Bruce-Smith, Alex. (2017, May 11). "15% of the Australian Population Is Now on Tinder." Pedestrian. https://www.pedestrian.tv/news/15-of-the-australian-population-is-now-on-tinder/

Bruckman, Amy. (1996). "Gender Swapping on the Internet." In *High Noon on the Electronic Frontier: Conceptual Issues in Cyberspace*, edited by Peter Ludlow, 317–326. Cambridge, MA: MIT Press.

Bryden, Lindsey T. (2017). "Online Dating Applications and the Uses and Gratifications Theory." https://dc.ewu.edu/cgi/viewcontent.cgi?article=1451&context=theses

Buchbinder, David. (2001). "Past and Future Tense: The Crisis in Masculinity." The Future of Gender Research Workshop. Retrieved April 28, 2005, from http://www.ias.uwa.edu.au/_data/page/17737/buchbinder.htm

Bumble. n.d. "Make the First Move." *Bumble*. Accessed 19 July 2021. https://bumble.com/en/about.

Bumble. (2017). "Press Kit." https://www.dropbox.com/sh/c17d9q0quyj59rw/AABkP-4jMOYLvXbeEkwbFJWnSa?dl=0 (February 7, 2018).

Butera, Karina J. (2008). "'Neo-mateship' in the 21st Century: Changes in the Performance of Australian Masculinity." *Journal of Sociology* 44 (3): 265–281. DOI: 10.1177/1440783308092884.

Butler, Judith. (1990). *Gender Trouble: Feminism and the Subversion of Identity*. New York: Routledge.

Bye Felipe (2021). "Instagram." https://www.instagram.com/byefelipe/?hl=en

Callon, Michel. (1986). "The Sociology of an Actor-Network: The Case of the Electric Vehicle." In *Mapping the Dynamics of Science and Technology*, edited by M. Callon, J. Law, and A. Rip. London: Palgrave Macmillan. DOI: 10.1007/978-1-349-07408-2_2

Can Australians Feel Love? Tumblr thread, 2014, captured here: https://ifunny.co/picture/no-lts-too-hot-to-feel-anything-when-our-neighbor-wHk9VRN556)'

Carlson, Bronwyn. (2020a). Love and hate at the cultural interface: indigenous Australians and dating Apps. *Journal of Sociology* 56 (2): 133–150.

Carlson, Bronwyn. (2020b). "Slow Love Podcast Series, Episode 17." https://www.slowlove.net/episodes/episode17-bronwyn

Carlson, Bronwyn, and Ryan Frazer (2018). "Cyberbullying and Indigenous Australians: A Review of the Literature." Aboriginal Health and Medical Research Council of New South Wales and Macquarie University, Sydney.

Cefai, Sarah, and Nick Couldry. (2017). "Mediating the Presence of Others: Reconceptualising Co-Presence as Mediated Intimacy." *SAGE Journals*. DOI: 10.1177/1367549417743040

Clemente-Suárez, Vicente Javier, Athanasios A. Dalamitros, Ana Isabel Beltran-Velasco, Juan Mielgo-Ayuso and Jose Francisco Tornero-Aguilera. (2020). "Social and Psychophysiological Consequences of the COVID-19 Pandemic: An Extensive Literature Review." *Frontiers in Psychology*. 11: 580225. DOI: 10.3389/fpsyg.2020.580225

Communiello, Francesca, Lorenza Parisi, and Francesca Ieracitano. (2020). "Negotiating Gender Scripts in Mobile Dating Apps: Between Affordances, Usage Norms and Practices." *Information, Communications and Society*. DOI: 10.1080/1369118x.2020.1787485

Condie, Jenna, Garth Lean and Donna James. (2018). "Tinder Matters: Swiping Right to Unlock New Research Fields." In *Doing Research in and on the Digital: Research Methods across Fields of Inquiry*, edited by Cristina Cosa and Jenna Condie, 102–115. London: Routledge.

Connell, B. (1995). *Masculinities.* Crows Nest: Allen & Unwin.

Connell, B., T. Carrigan, and J. Lee. (2001). "Toward a New Sociology of Masculinity." In *The Masculinity Studies Reader*, edited by R. Adams and D. Savran, 99–117. Oxford: Blackwell.

Conner, Christopher T. (2019). "The Gay Gayze: Expressions of Inequality on Grindr." *The Sociological Quarterly* 60: 397–419.

Consalvo, Mia. (2003). "Hot Dates and Fairy-Tale Romances: Studying Sexuality in Video Games." In *The Video Game Theory Reader Mark*, edited by J. P. Wolf and Bernard Perron, 171–194. London: Routledge.

Coole, Diana, and Samantha Frost. (2010). *New Materialisms: Ontology, Agency and Politics.* Durham, NC: Duke University Press. DOI: 10.1215/9780822392996

Cyr, Jennifer. (2017). "The Unique Utility of Focus Groups for Mixed-Methods Research." *PS: Political Science and Politics* 50 (4): 1038–1042. DOI: 10.1017/S104909651700024X

David, Gaby, and Carolina Cambre. (2016). "Screened Intimacies: Tinder and the Swipe Logic." *Social Media and Society* 2 (2): published first online. DOI: 10.1177/2056305116641976.

De Laurentis, Teresa. (1993). "Sexual Indifference and Lesbian Representation." In *The Gay and Lesbian Studies Reader*, edited by H. Abelove, M. Barale, and D. Haperin, 141–158. New York: Routledge.

Department of Health (2020). Physical Distancing (explainer vide0). https://www.health.gov.au/resources/videos/coronavirus-covid-19-video-physical-distancing

Deterding, Sebastian, Dan Dixon, Rilla Khaled, and Lennart Nacke. (2011). "From Game Design Elements to Gamefulness: Defining "gamification"." MindTrek'11: Proceedings of the 15th International Academic MindTrek Conference: Envisioning Future Media Environments. September 2011, pp. 9–15. DOI: 10.1145/2181037.2181040

Di Maggio, Paul, and Estzer Hargittai. (2001). "From the Digital Divide to Digital Inequity: Studying Internet Use as Penetration Increases." Centre for Arts and Cultural Studies, Princeton.

Dietzel, Christopher, David Myles, and Stefanie Duguay. (2021). "Relationships during a Pandemic: How Dating Apps have Adapted to COVID-19." The Conversation. https://theconversation.com/relationships-during-a-pandemic-how-dating-apps-have-adapted-to-covid-19-160219

Dixson, Miriam. (1999). *The Real Matilda: Woman and Identity in Australia, 1788 to the Present.* Sydney: UNSW Press.

Doherty, Thomas. (2010). "The Rom-Com Genre and the Shopping Gene." *OAH Magazine of History* 24 (2): 25–28. DOI: 10.1093/maghis/24.2.25.

Domonoske, Camila. (2018). "The Tinder Bumble Feud: Dating Apps Fight over Who Owns the Swipe, npr." https://www.npr.org/2018/10/30/660006488/the-tinder-bumble-feud-dating-apps-fight-over-who-owns-the-swipe

Doty, Nathan D., Brian L. Willoughby, Kristin M. Lindahl, and Neena M. Malik. (2010 October). "Sexuality Related Social Support among Lesbian, Gay, and Bisexual Youth." *Journal of Youth and Adolescence* 39 (10): 1134–1147. DOI: 10.1007/s10964-010-9566-x. Epub 2010 Jul 1. PMID: 20593304.

Duguay, Stefanie. (2016). "Lesbian, Gay, Bisexual, Trans and Queer Visibility through selfies: comparing platform mediators across Ruby Rose's Instagram and Vine Presence." *Social Media and Society.* 2(2): 1–12. DOI: 10.1177/2056305116641975.

Duguay, Stefanie. (2017). "Dressing up Tinderella: Interrogating Authenticity Claims on the Mobile Dating App Tinder." *Information, Communication & Society* 20 (3): 351–367. DOI: 10.1080/1369118X.2016.1168471.

Duguay, Stefanie. (2017). "You Can't Use this App for That: Exploring Off-Label Use through an Investigation of Tinder." *The Information Society* 36 (1): 30–42. DOI: 10.1080/01972243.2019.1685036.

Elder, Catriona. (2020). *Being Australian: Narratives of National Identity.* Abingdon: Routledge.

Ferris, Lindsay, and Stefanie Duguay. (2019). "Tinder's Lesbian Digital Imaginary: Investigating (im)permeable Boundaries of Sexual Identity on a Popular Dating App." *New Media & Society* 22 (3): 489–506. Article first published online: July 24, 2019; Issue published: March 1, 2020. DOI: 10.1177/1461444819864903

Fetters, Ashley. (2018, December 21). "The Five Years That Changed Dating." The Atlantic. https://www.theatlantic.com/family/archive/2018/12/tinder-changed-dating/578698/

Fetters, Ashley and Kaitlyn Tiffany. (2020). "The 'Dating Market' is Getting Worse." *The Atlantic*, 26 February. Accessed 19 July 2021. https://www.theatlantic.com/family/archive/2020/02/modern-dating-odds-economy-apps-tinder-math/606982/

Firestone, Shulamith. (1970). *The Diabetic of Sex.* New York: William Morrow and Company.

Foubert, John D., Matthew W. Brosi, & R. Sean Bannon (2011). "Pornography Viewing among Fraternity Men: Effects on Bystander Intervention, Rape Myth Acceptance and Behavioral Intent to Commit Sexual Assault." *Sexual Addiction & Compulsivity* 18 (4): 212–231. DOI: 10.1080/10720162.2011.625552

Fox, Nick J., and Pam Alldred. (2017). "Sociology and the New Materialism: Theory, Research, Action." SAGE Publication Ltd. DOI: 10.4135/9781526401915

Freier, A. (2015). *Tinder Mobile App Statistics and Revenue.* Accessed 22 September 2015. http://www.businessofapps.com/tinder-mobile-app-statistics-and-revenue/

Freitas, Donna. (2013). *The End of Sex: How Hookup Culture Is Leaving a Generation Unhappy, Sexually Unfulfilled, and Confused about Intimacy.* New York: Basic Books.

Fullagar, Simone, Emma Rich, Jessica Francombe-Webb, and Antonio Maturo. (2017). "Digital Ecologies of Youth Mental Health: Apps, Therapeutic Publics and Pedagogy as Affective Arrangements." *Social Sciences* 6: 135. 10.3390/socsci6040135.

Gagnon, John H. (1990). "The Explicit and Implicit Use of the Scripting Perspective in Sex Research." *Annual Review of Sex Research* 1 (1): 1–43. DOI: 10.1080/10532528.1990.10559854.

Gagnon, John H., and William Simon. (1973). *Sexual Conduct: The Social Sources of Human Sexuality.* Chicago, IL: Aldine.

Gebel, Meira. (2019, February 11). "I'm 25, and I Talked to 3 Single Women in Their 50s about What It's Like to Use Dating Apps Like Tinder and Bumble." Their experiences surprised Sme. Business Insider. https://www.businessinsider.com.au/older-women-dating-apps-experiences-tinder-bumble-2019-2?r=US&IR=T

Giddens, Anthony. (1991). *Modernity and Self-Identity: Self and Society in the Late Modern Age.* Cambridge: Polity.

Giddens, Anthony. (1992). *The Transformation of Intimacy: Sexuality, Love, and Eroticism in Modern Societies.* Stanford: Stanford University Press.

Gill, Rosalind, and Akane Kanai. (2018). "Mediating Neoliberal Capitalism: Affect, Subjectivity and Inequality." *Journal of Communication* 68: 318–326.

Goffman, Erving. (1990). *The Presentation of Self in Everyday Life (1959).* London: Penguin.

Grauerholtz, Elizabeth, and Richard T. Serpe. (1985). "Initiation and Response: The Dynamics of Sexual Interaction." *Sex Roles* 12 (9): 1041–1059. DOI: 10.1007/BF00288104.

Griffin, Christine. (2004). "Good Girls, Bad Girls: Anglocentrism and Diversity in the Constitution of Contemporary Girlhood." In *All about the Girl: Culture, Power and Identity*, edited by Anita Harris, 29–44. New York: Routledge

Grindon, Leger. (2011). *The Hollywood Romantic Comedy: Conventions, History, Controversies*. Wiley Online.

Grosz, Elizabeth. (1994). *Volatile Bodies: Toward a Corporeal Feminism*. Sydney: Allen & Unwin.

Hakala, Kate. (2015). "This Is Why Men Outnumber Women Two-to-One on Tinder." MIC. https://www.mic.com/articles/110774/two-thirds-of-tinder-users-are-men-here-s-whyd

Hanson, Kenneth R. (2021). "Collective Exclusion: How White Heterosexual Dating App Norms Reproduce Status Quo Hookup Culture." *Sociological Inquiry*, published ahead of print. DOI: 10.1111/soin.12426.

Hartmann, Heidi I. (1981). "The Family as the Locus of Gender, Class, and Political Struggle: The Example of Housework." *Signs* 6: 366–394.

Heale, Roberta, and Alison Twycross. (2020). "What Is a Case Study?" *Evidenced Based Nursing*. https://ebn.bmj.com/content/21/1/7#aff-1

Heldman, Caroline. (2010). "Hook-up Culture: Setting a New Research Agenda." *Sexuality Research and Social Policy*. DOI: 10.1007/s13178-010-0024-z

Helsper, Ellen, and Monica Whitty. (2010). "Netiquette within Married Couples: Agreement about Acceptable Online Behavior and Surveillance between Partners." *Computers in Human Behavior* 26 (5): 916–926. ISSN 0747–5632

Hess, Aaron, and Carlos Flores. (2018). "Simply More Than Swiping Left: A Critical Analysis of Toxic Masculine Performances on Tinder Nightmares." *New Media & Society* 20: 1085–1102.

Hobbs, Mitchell, Stephen Owen, and Livia Gerber. (2016). "Liquid Love? Dating Apps, Sex, Relationships and the Digital Transformation of Intimacy." *Journal of Sociology* 53 (2): 271–284. DOI: 10.1177/1440783316662718.

Hobdey, Liz. (2020). "Older Men Charged More for Using Tinder's Premium Service, Choice Mystery Shoppers Find." https://www.abc.net.au/news/2020-08-12/tinder-price-setting-more-expensive-for-older-people-looking-to/12549186

Huang, Evelyn T., Henrietta Williams, Jane S. Hocking, and Megan S. C. Lim (2016). "Safe Sex Messages within Dating and Entertainment Smartphone Apps: A Review." *JMIR MHealth and UHealth* 4 (4). Available from: https://mhealth.jmir.org/2016/4/e124/. DOI: 10.2196/mhealth.5760.

Ibal, Mansoor. (2021). "Tinder Revenue and Usage Statistics (2021)." Business of Apps, https://www.businessofapps.com/data/tinder-statistics/

Illouz, Eva. (1997). *Consuming the Romantic Utopia: Love and the Cultural Contradictions of Capitalism*. Berkeley: University of California Press.

Illouz, Eva. (2013). *Why Love Hurts: A Sociological Explanation*. Oxford: John Wiley and Sons. ISBN: 978-0-745-67107-9

Illouz, Eva. (2009). "Emotions, Imagination and Consumption: A new research agenda." *Journal of Consumer Culture* 9 (3): 377–413. DOI: 10.1177/1469540509342053

Irigaray, Luce. (1974). *Speculum of the Other Woman*. Ithaca, NY: Cornell University Press.

Irigaray, Luce. (1979). *This Sex Which Is Not One*. Ithaca, NY: Cornell University Press.

Jamieson, Lynn and Hedvig Ekerwald. (1998). *Intimacy. Personal Relationships in Modern Societies*. Cambridge: Polity.

Jamieson, L. (2013). "Personal Relationships, Intimacy and the Self in a Mediated and Global Digital Age." In *Digital Sociology: Critical Perspectives*, edited by Kate Orton-Johnson and Nicholas Prior. Palgrave Macmillan. DOI: 10.1057/9781137297792_2

Joost, Henry, and Ariel Schulman. (2010). *Catfish*. https://pro.imdb.com/title/tt1584016/?rf=cons_tt_atf&ref_=cons_tt_atf

Junkee. (2020, October). "Absolutely Sickening: Australians Are Shocked by Tinder's Response to Sexual Assault." https://junkee.com/4-corners-tinder-sexual-assault-hack-reactions/274164

Kanai, Akane. (2017). "The Best Friend, the Boyfriend, Other Girls, Hot Guys, and Creeps: The Relational Production of Self on Tumblr." *Feminist Media Studies* 17 (6): 911–925. DOI: 10.1080/14680777.2017.1298647

Kermode, Frank. (1970). *The Genesis of Secrecy: On the Interpretation of Narrative*. Cambridge, MA: Harvard University Press.

Kincaid, Jason. (2009, March 25). "Gay Dating Makes Its Way to the iPhone." TechCrunch. https://techcrunch.com/2009/03/25/gay-dating-makes-its-way-to-the-iphone/

Kivel, B. Dana, and Corey W. Johnson. (2009). "Consuming Media, Making Men: Using Collective Memory Work to Understand Leisure and the Construction of Masculinity." *Journal of Leisure Research* 41 (1): 110–134.

Knight, Jamie. (2020). *Cramped Quarters: An Enemies to Lovers Accidental Roommates Romance*. Self-published.

Kosoff, Maya. (2014). "Report: Ousted Tinder Cofounder Settled Her Sexual Harassment Lawsuit against the Company for Just Over 1 Million." Business Insider. https://www.businessinsider.com.au/whitney-wolfe-settles-sexual-harassment tinder-lawsuit-1-million-2014-11

Krieg, Hannah. (2020). "100 Percent Feminist': Is Bumble More Than a Gimmick?" The Daily. https://www.dailyuw.com/wellness/article_d70aba3c-9352-11ea-a278-e3d7e9c4671f.html

Kupers, Terry A. (2005). "Toxic Masculinity as a Barrier to Mental Health Treatment in Prison." *Journal of Clinical Psychology* 61: 713–724.

Lauckner, Carolyn, Danielle Lambert, Natalia Truszczynski, and Nathan Hansen. (2021). Dating App Use among Rural Men Who Have Sex with Men and Its Relationship to HIV Prevention and Risk Behaviors: A Mixed-Methods Analysis." *Rural Remote Health*. DOI: 10.22605/RRH6556

Lee, Jin. (2019). "Mediated Superficiality and Misogyny Mediated through cool on Tinder." *SAGE Journal*. DOI: 10.1177/2056305119872949

Lehmiller, Justin J., and Michael Loerger. (2014, January 23). "Social Networking Smartphone Applications and Sexual Health Outcomes among Men Who Have Sex with Men." *PLoS One* 9 (1): e86603. DOI: 10.1371/journal.pone.0086603. PMID: 24466166; PMCID: PMC3900560.

Levy, Ariel. (2010). *Female Chauvinist Pigs: Women and the Rise of Raunch Culture*. New York: Free Press.

Lewis, Tom. (1994). "The Politics of "Hauntology" in Derrida's Specters of Marx. Rethinking Marxism." *A Journal of Economics, Culture and Society* 9, 1996 (3), 64.

Liamputtong, Pranee. (2007). *Researching the Vulnerable: A Guide to Sensitive Research Methods*. Thousand Oaks, CA: SAGE.

Liau, Adrian, Gregorio Millett, and Gary Marks. (2006). "Meta-Analytic Examination of Online Sex-Seeking and Sexual Risk Behvaior among Men Who Have Sex with Men." *Journal of Sex and Trans Men*. DOI: 10.1097/01.olq.0000204710.35332.c5

Liddy, Matt, and Cristen Tilley. (2020, December 10). "Four Australia Talks Findings That Can Help Us Understand 2020." ABC. https://www.abc.net.au/news/2020-12-10/australia-talks-findings-2020-insights/12955570

Lin, Melissa. (2018). "Online Dating Industry: The Business of Love." https://www.toptal.com/finance/business-model-consultants/online-dating-industry. Finance online.

Lupton, Deborah. (2018). "How Do Data Come to Matter? Living and Becoming with Personal Data." *SAGE Journals*. DOI: 10.1177/2053951718786314

Lupton, Deborah. (2019). "Towards a More-Than-Human Analysis of Digital Health." Part 2, Chapter *Pearls, Pith and Provocation*. London: Sage.

Macapagal, Kathryn, David A. Moskowitz, Dennis H. Li, Andrés Carrión, Emily Bettin, Celia B. Fisher, and Brian Mustanski. (2018). "Hookup App Use, Sexual Behavior, and Sexual Health among Adolescent Men Who Have Sex with Men in the United States." *Journal of Adolescent Health* 62 (6): 708–715. ISSN 1054–139X. DOI: 10.1016/j.jadohealth.2018.01.001.

Macleod, Caitlin, and Victoria McArthur. (2018). "The Construction of Gender in DatingApps: An Interface Analysis of Tinder and Bumble." *Feminist Media Studies* 19 (6): 922–940. DOI: 10.1080/14680777.2018.1494618.

Mamamia. (2018). "A Man Asked for a Pic of My Armpits. But What He Did Next Was Most Unnerving." https://www.mamamia.com.au/tinder-messages-online-dating/

Matamoros-Fernandez, Ariadna. (2017). "Platformed Racism: The Mediation and Circulation of an Australian Race-Based Controversy on Twitter, Facebook and YouTube." 930–946.

McAlister, Jodi. (2018a). "The Literary Text as Historical Artifact: The Colonial Couple in Australian Romantic Fiction by Women, 1838–60." *Lilith* 24: 38–51.

McAlister, Jodi. (2018b). "'Feelings like the women in books': Declarations of Love in Australian Romance Novels, 1859–1891." *Emotions: History, Culture, Society* 2 (1): 91–112. DOI: 10.1163/2208522X-02010005.

McAlister, Jodi. (2020). The *Consummate Virgin: Female Virginity Loss and Love in Anglophone Popular Literatures*. Cham: Palgrave.

McAlister, Jodi, and Hsu-Ming Teo. (2017) "Love in Australian Romance Novels." In *The Popular Culture of Romantic Love in Australia*, edited by Hsu-Ming Teo, 194–222. Melbourne: Australian Scholarly Publishing.

McDonald, Tamar J. (2007). *Romantic Comedy: Boy Meets Girl Meets Genre*. New York: Columbia University Press.

McGlotten, Shaka. (2013). *Virtual Intimacies: Media, Affect, and Queer Sociality*. Albany, NY: SUNY Press.

McIntosh, Michele J., and Janice M. Morse. (2015). "Situating and Constructing Diversity in Semi-Structured Interviews." *Global Qualitative Nursing Research*, First Published August 14, 2015 Research Article Find in PubMed. DOI: 10.1177/2333393615597674

McLaren, Angus. (1999). *Twentieth-Century Sexuality: A History*. Oxford: Blackwell.

McNeill, Patrick, et al. (2005). *Research Methods*. London: Routledge. ISBN 9780415340762

McRobbie, Angela. (1997). "Bridging the Gap: Feminism, Fashion and Consumption." *Feminist Review* 55, 73–89.

McRobbie, Angela. (2009). *The Aftermath of Feminism: Gender, Culture and Social Change*. Oxford: SAGE.

Ménard, A. Dana, and Christine Cabrera. (2011). "'Whatever the Approach: Tab B Still Fits into Slot A': Twenty Years of Sex Scripts in Romance Novels." *Sexuality and Culture* 15: 240–255. DOI: 10.1007/s12119-011-9092-3.

Meyers, Nancy. (Directer). (2006). The Holiday. Columbia Pictures.

Mitchell, Kimberly, David Finkelhor, Lisa Jones, and Janis Wolak. (2011). "Prevalence and Characteristics of Youth Sexting: A National Study." *Pediatrics* 129: 13–20. DOI: 10.1542/peds.2011-1730.

Mori, Camille, Jeff R. Temple, Dillon Browne, and Sheri Madigan. (2019, August 1). "Association of Sexting with Sexual Behaviors and Mental Health among Adolescents:

A Systematic Review and Meta-analysis." *JAMA Pediatrics*. 173 (8): 770–779. DOI: 10.1001/jamapediatrics.2019.1658. PMID: 31206151; PMCID: PMC6580450.

Mruck, Katja, and Gunter Mey. (2019). "Grounded Theory Methodology and Self-Reflexivity in the Qualitative Research Process." In *The SAGE Handbook of Current Developments in Grounded Theory*, 470–496. SAGE Publications Ltd. DOI: 10.4135/9781526485656

Murphy, Kristina, et al. (2020, June 30). "Coronavirus Spike: Why Getting People to Follow Restrictions Is Harder the Second Time around." The Conversation. https://theconversation.com/coronavirus-spike-why-getting-people-to-follow-restrictions-is-harder-the-second-time-around-141287

Murrie, Linzi. (1998). "The Australian Legend: Writing Australian Masculinity / Writing 'Australian' Masculine." *Journal of Australian Studies* 22 (56): 68–77. DOI: 10.1080/14443059809387361.

Newett, Lyndsay, Brendan Churchill, and Brady Robards. (2017). "Forming Connections in the Digital Era: Tinder, a New Tool in Young Australian Intimate Life." *Journal of Sociology* 54. DOI: 10.1177/1440783317728584.

Neuman, Russell. (2010). *Media, Technology and Society – Theories of Media Evolution*. Ann Arbor: The University of Michigan Press.

news.com. (2020, October). "Tinder Ignored Reports of Raps as Offenders Exploit Dating App." https://www.news.com.au/technology/online/internet/four-corners-tinder-ignored-reports-of-rape-as-offenders-exploit-dating-app/news-story/67421b447114a804d6f07c91140f5b17

news.com. (2020). "Why Tinder Is the Sleaziest Dating App." https://www.news.com.au/lifestyle/relationships/dating/why-tinder-is-the-sleaziest-online-dating-app/news-story/db79daec79229ba4c407388bd81a02d2

Ng, Alfred. (2019). "Cyberstalkers are Crowdsourcing Danger to Victims' Doorsteps with Dating Apps." *CNet*, 23 January. Accessed 19 July 2021. https://www.cnet.com/news/cyberstalkers-are-crowdsourcing-danger-to-victims-doorsteps-with-dating-apps/

Patel, Nilay, and Ashley Carman. (2020, June 9). "Tinder CEO Elie Seidman on Finding Love during the Pandemic." The Verge. https://www.theverge.com/21284420/tinder-ceo-elie-seidman-interview-dating-pandemic

Peterson, Anne H. (2014b, February 28). "Jennifer Lawrence and the History of Cool Girls." *Buzzfeed News*. Retrieved from https://www.buzzfeed.com/annehelen-petersen/jennifer-lawrence-and-the-history-of-cool-girls?utm_term=.siK884Aed#.iaqqqy0lX

Paul, Gerd, and Christian Stegbauer. (2005). "Is the Digital Divide between Young and Elderly People Increasing?" *First Monday* 10 (10). DOI: 10.5210/fm.v10i10.1286

Pingel, Emily S., Jose A. Bauermeister, Michelle M. Johns, Anna Eisenberg, and MatthewLeslie-Santana. (2013). "'A Safe Way to Explore': Reframing Risk on the Internet amidst Young Gay Men's Search for Identity." 28 (4): 453–478. Article first published online: February 25, 2013; Issue published: July 1, 2013. DOI: 10.1177/0743558412470985

Plant, Sadie. (1997). *Zeros and Ones*. London: Fourth Estate.

Pond, Tara, and Panteá Farvid. (2017). "'I do like girls, I promise': Young Bisexual Women's Experiences of Using Tinder." *Psychology of Sexualities Review* 8 (2): 6–24.

Portolan, Lisa, and Jodi McAlister. (2021). "Jagged Love: Narratives of Romance on Dating Apps during COVID-19." *Sexuality & Culture*, forthcoming.

Radway, Janice. (1984). *Reading the Romance: Women, Patriarchy and Popular Literature*. University of North Carolina Press.

Rao, Leena. (2011, March 31). "Exclusive: IAC Hatches Hatch Labs, a Technology Sandbox to Incubate Mobile Startups." TechCrunch. https://techcrunch.com/2011/03/31/exclusive-iac-hatches-hatch-a-technology-sandbox-to-incubate-mobile-startups/

Regis, Pamela. (2003). *A Natural History of the Romance Novel*. Philadelphia: University of Pennsylvania Press.

Reid, Elizabeth. (1996). "Text-Based Virtual Realities: Identity and the Cyborg Body." In *High Noon on the Electronic Frontier: Conceptual Issues in Cyberspace*, edited by Peter Ludlow, 317–326. Cambridge, MA: MIT Press.

Reilly, Andrew, and Eirik J. Saethre (2013). "The Hankie Code Revisited: From Function to Fashion." *Critical Studies in Men's Fashion* 1 (1): 69–78.

Renninger, Bryce J. (2018). "Grindr Killed the Gay Bar, and Other Attempts to Blame Social Technologies for Urban Development: A Democratic Approach to Popular Technologies and Queer Sociality." *Journal of Homosexuality*. DOI: 10.1080/00918369.2018.1514205

Ricoeur, Paul. (1990). *Time and Narrative*, vol. 1. (K. McLaughlin & D. Pellauer, Trans.). Chicago, IL: Chicago University Press.

Ringrose, Jessica, and Amy S. Dobson. (2015). "Sext Education: Pedagogies of Sex, Gender and Shame in the Schoolyards of Tagged and Exposed." *Sex Education*. DOI: 10.1080/14681811.2015.1050486

Robards, Brady, and Siân Lincoln. (2017). "Uncovering Longitudinal Life Narratives: Scrolling Back on Facebook." *Qualitative Research* 17 (6): 715–730. DOI: 10.1177/1468794117700707

Roche, Gerald, Hiroshi Maruyama, and Åsa V. Kroik. (2018). *Indigenous Efflorescence: Beyond Revitalisation in Sapmi and Ainu Mosir*. Canberra: ANU Press.

Roseneil, Sasha, et al. (2020). *The Tenacity of the Couple-Norm: Intimate Citizenship Regimes in a Changing Europe*. London: UCL Press.

Sales, Nancy J. (2015, August 6). "Tinder and the Dawn of the "dating apocalypse"." Vanity Fair. Retrieved from www.vanityfair.com/culture/2015/08/tinder-hook-up-culture-end-of-dating

Saraiva, Luiz Alex Silva, Leonardo Tadeu dos Santos, and Jefferson Rodrigues Perreira. (2020). "Heteronormativity, Masculinity and Prejudice in Mobile Apps: The Case of Grindr in a Brazilian City." *Brazilian Business Review* 17 (1): 114–131. DOI: 10.15728/bbr.2020.17.1.6.

Schreurs, Lara, Sindy R. Sumter, and Laura Vandenbosch. (2020). "A Prototype Willingness Approach to the Relation between Geo-social Dating Apps and Willingness to Sext with Dating App Matches." *Archives of Sexual Behavior* 49 (4): 1133–1145. DOI: 10.1007/s10508-020-01671-5. Epub 2020 Mar 13. PMID: 32170549.

Seidman, Elie. (2020). "On the Verge. Tinder CEO Elie Seidman on Finding Love during the Pandemic." https://www.theverge.com/21284420/tinder-ceo-elie-seidman-interview-dating-pandemic

Shield, Andrew. (2017). ""Looking for North Europeans Only": Identifying Five Racist Patterns in an Online Subculture." *Kult-Postkolonial Temaserie* 15: 87–106.

Shildrick, Margrit. (1997). *Leaky Bodies and Boundaries: Feminism, Postmodernism and (bio) ethics*. London: Routledge.

Shumway, David. (2003). *Modern Love: Romance, Intimacy, and the Marriage Crisis*. New York: NYU Press.

Simon, William, and John H. Gagnon. (1986). "Sexual Scripts: Permanence and Change." *Archives of Sexual Behavior* 15 (2): 97–120. DOI: 10.1007/BF01542219.

Simon, William, and John H. Gagnon. (1987). "A Sexual Scripts Approach." In *Theories of Human Sexuality*, edited by James H. Geer and William T. O'Donohue, 363–383. New York: Plenum Press.

Simon, William, and John H. Gagnon. (2003). "Sexual Scripts: Origins, Influences and Changes." *Qualitative Sociology* 26 (4): 491–497. DOI: 10.1023/B:QUAS.0000005053.99846.e5.

Smith, Christian. (2011). *Lost in Transition: The Dark Side of Emerging Adulthood.* Oxford University Press. https://doi.org/10.1093/acprof:oso/9780199828029.003.0002

Stephure, Robert J., Susan D. Boon, Stacey L. MacKinnon, and Vicki L. Deveau. (2009). "Internet Initiated Relationships: Associations between Age and Involvement in Online Dating." *Journal of Computer-Mediated Communication* 14 (3): 658–681. DOI: 10.1111/j.1083-6101.2009.01457.x

Suchman, Lucy. (2007). *Human-Machine Reconfigurations: Plans and Situated Actions.* Cambridge: Cambridge University Press.

Taylor, Anthea. (2008). *Mediating Australian Feminism.* Oxford: Peter Lang.

Taylor, Anthea. (2012). *Single Women in Popular Culture.* Oxford: Peter Lang.

The Age. (2002). "Changing the Game." The Age. https://www.theage.com.au/lifestyle/changing-the-game-20120211-1sy90.html#ixzz1mTfkGD2D

The Conversation. (2017). "Terrorist or Hipster – What Does a Beard Mean?" https://theconversation.com/terrorist-or-hipster-what-does-a-beard-mean-74251

The Conversation. (August, 2021). "Man to Face Court over Alleged Rape of Brittany Higgins." https://theconversation.com/man-to-face-court-over-alleged-rape-of-brittany-higgins-165763

The Daily Mail. (2018). "Dating App Giant Tinder Sues Rival Bumble." https://www.dailymail.co.uk/news/article-5514717/Dating-app-giant-Tinder-sues-rival-Bumble.html

The Guardian. (2019). "Dating Apps: Has Tinder Lost Its Spark." https://www.theguardian.com/technology/2019/aug/11/dating-apps-has-tinder-lost-its-spark

Thompson, Laura. (2018). ""I Can Be Your Tinder Nightmare": Harassment and Misogyny in the Online Sexual Marketplace." *Feminism & Psychology* 28: 69–89.

Thompson, Rachel. (2019, June 7). "In the Dating Game, Women Are Pressured to Play the Part of a Stereotypical "cool girl"." Mashable. Retrieved from https://mashable.com/article/cool-girl-stereotype-dating-culture/?europe=true

Tinder. n.d. "So, Why Choose a Dating App Like Tinder?" *Tinder.* Accessed 19 July 2021. https://tinder.com/about-tinder.

TinderNightmares. (2021). Instagram. https://www.instagram.com/tindernightmares/?hl=en

Toma, Catalina L., Jeffrey T. Hancock, and Nicole B. Ellison. (2008). "Separating Fact from Fiction: An Examination of Deceptive Self-Presentation in Online Dating." *Personality and Social Psychology Bulletin* 34: 1023–1036.

Toma, Catalina L., L. Crystal Jiang, and Jeffrey T. Hancock. (2018). "Lies in the Eye of the Beholder: Asymmetric Beluefs about One's Own and Others' Deceptiveness in Mediated and Face-to-Face Communication." *Communication Research* 45 (8): 1167–1192.

Tomaszewska, Paulina, and Isabell Schuster. (2020). "Comparing Sexuality-Related Cognitions Sexual Behaviour and Acceptance of Sexual Coercion in Dating App Users and Non-Users." *Sexuality Research and Social Policy* 17: 188–198. DOI: 10.1007/s13178-019-00397-x

Tse-Shang Tang, Denise. (2017). "All I Get Is an Emoji: Dating on Lesbian Mobile Phone App Butterfly." 39 (6): 816–832. Article first published online: March 6, 2017; Issue published: September 1, 2017. DOI: 10.1177/0163443717693680

Vincent, Louise, and Caryn McEwen. (2004). "Sleeping with Beauty: Romantic Love, Sex, Power and the Construction of Femininity in Heterosexual Young Adult Relationships." *Asian Women* 20: 1–26.

Waling, Andrea. (2019). *White Masculinity in Contemporary Australia: The Good Ol' Aussie Bloke*. Abingdon: Routledge.

Whitman, Kirsty W. (2013). Looking out for the Aussie Bloke: Gender, Class and Contextualising a Hegemony of the Working-Class Masculinities in Australia, submitted for PhD.

Whitty, Monica, and Tom Buchanan. (2015). "The Online Dating Romance Scam: The Psychological Impact on Victims – Both Financial and Non-Financial." *Criminology and Criminal Justice*. DOI: 10.1177/1748895815603773

Wiegman, Robyn. (1995). *American Anatomies: Theorizing Race and Gender*. Durham, NC: Duke University Press.

Wikipedia, "Grindr" (app) (last updated March 2021). https://en.wikipedia.org/wiki/Grindr

Wikipedia, "Tinder" (app) (last updated March 2021). https://en.wikipedia.org/wiki/Tinder_(app)

Wikipedia, "Whitney Wolfe Herd" (last updated March 2021). https://en.wikipedia.org/wiki/Whitney_Wolfe_Herd

Winch, Alison. (2013). *Girlfriends and Postfeminist Sisterhood*. Basingstoke: Palgrave.

Yashari, Leora. (2015, August 7). "Meet the Tinder Co-Founder Trying to Change Online Dating Forever." Vanity Fair. http://www.vanityfair.com/culture/2015/08/bumble-app-whitney-wolfe (February 6, 2018).

YouGov. (2017). "A Third of Aussies Have Used Internet Dating." *YouGov*, 23 November. Accessed 19 July 2021. https://au.yougov.com/news/2017/11/23/internet-dating/

YouGov. (2019). "Internet Dating." https://au.yougov.com/news/2017/11/23/internet-dating/

INDEX

Aapola, Sinikka 59
Albury, Kath 11, 76
Andreev, Andre 16, 17
animation 42, 44, 49, 85
anxiety: around romantic relationships/ milestones 29–31, 74–75, 78–82, 88; busy-ness and 35, 49–50, 78, 83, 88; COVID-19 and 22–24; use of romantic masterplot(s) in response to 25–26, 37
Aussie Bloke stereotype: desirability and 53, 86; facial/body hair and 55, 86–87; as highly gendered 53–54, 86–87; inability of ethnically diverse to men to conform to 51, 55–56, 87; misogynistic overtones of 54; physicality of 54–55; relationship prospects and 57–58; self-worth and 51–52, 87; subversion of 64; toxic masculinity and 58–59, 65, 87; updates to 55, 64, 87
authenticity 61–62

Badoo 17
Bartky, Sandra Lee 60
Battersby, Michelle 18
Bauman, Zygmunt 6, 20–21, 31, 34, 37, 40, 64
Beck, Ulrich 40
Belsey, Catherine 33
Berlant, Lauren 7, 32, 38–39, 44, 66, 72, 74, 84
biocommunicability theory 11
Bivens, Rena 15–16
body hair 55, 86–87
Boellstorff, Tom 4–5
bogan term 56
Bowers, Jack 54
branding concept 59–60, 64, 87
Brooks, Peter 6
Bumble: about 17–18; COVID-19 and 12–14, 22; as "female-focused," 14–18; functionality of 18–19; gender and 5, 14–17, 26; inaccessibility of to outsiders 8, 11, 76; Tinder and 16, 28; video chat and 13
busy-ness 34–35, 49–50, 78, 83, 88
Butera, Karina J. 54
Byron, Paul 11

Calvino, Italo 34–35
Carlson, Bronwyn 12
casual sex 30–31, 36–37, 84
celebrities 71–72, 75, 81
Chappy 18
chemistry 33–34, 85
Cheremkin, Max 18
Condie, Jenna 5, 15, 88
consensual non-monogamy 35–36, 82
COVID-19: consensual non-monogamy and 82; gender scripts and 52, 65–68; jagged love cycle and 74; media attention on dating apps and 12–14; mental health and 21–24; romantic masterplot(s) is response to anxiety from 25–26; romantic milestones and 74–75, 78–79; singles' bubbles and 22–23; Slow Love podcast and 69–70; surge in dating app

sign ups and 2, 22–24; time compression and 24–25, 70–71, 74–75, 77–78; video chats and 23

dating apps: busy-ness of 49–50, 78, 83, 88; chemistry and 33–34; consensual non-monogamy and 35–36, 82; COVID-19 and 2, 5–6, 8–9, 20–21, 23–24, 77–79; gender and 5, 25–26; geospatial aspect of 4–6; health concerns about 3; hook-up culture and 3, 20; hook-up vs. relationship-seeking profiles 28, 84; inaccessibility of to outsiders 8, 11, 76; intimacy and 7; jagged love concept and 6–7, 31–34, 37, 83, 85, 89; LGBTQ+ community and 4–5, 12, 75; Liquid Love concept and 6, 20–21, 27; meet-cute trope and 26–27; pandemic response of 12–13, 78; polarization of conversation about 7, 76; racism on 55–57, 68, 75, 89; romantic masterplot(s) and 4, 6–7, 36–37, 78–79, 88; safety concern reporting and 3, 9–12; self-worth and 41–42, 57, 64–65, 87; usage of in Australia 2–3; vulnerable communities and 12, 75
Dixson, Miriam 54
Doherty, Thomas 26
Duguay, Stefanie 5, 13, 15, 26

e-harmony 3
Elder, Catriona 54

Facebook 5, 26
facial hair 55, 86–87
Fahd, Cherine 55–56
FOMO (fear of missing out) 9, 14, 31, 34–35, 83

Gagnon, John H. 6
gender 5–6, 14–16, 25–26, 86; *see also* gender scripts
gender scripts: consultations with same-gender advisors 58, 62–63, 65, 87; COVID-19 and 52, 65–68; effort and 52; facial/body hair 55, 86–87; fear of intimidating prospects and 61; femininity scripts 51, 59–63, 65, 87–88; girlfriend culture and 63; gold digger stereotype and 73–74; heterosexiness and 58, 60–61, 65–66, 86; High-Maintenance Girl stereotype 51–52, 59–61, 67, 73–76; jagged love cycle and 52, 65, 67–68; LGBTQ+ community and 56–57; masculinity scripts 51, 53–59, 64–65, 86–87; othering and 51, 87; public relations language and 59–60, 64, 87; race and 55–57; self-worth and 57, 64–65, 87; subversion of 52, 64–65, 67; Tinder/Bumble functionality and 56, 86; toxic masculinity and 58–59, 65, 87; *see also* Aussie Bloke stereotype
Gerber, Livia 2
Giddens, Anthony 32, 38, 40, 44, 84
Gonick, Marnina 59
Griffin, Christine 60
Grindr 3, 5, 26, 56–57
Gulczynski, Chris 17

Hanson, Kenneth 5, 26
Harris, Anita 59
Hatch Labs 16
heteronormativity 4–5, 26–27, 63, 86
heterosexiness 58, 60–61, 65–66, 86
Higgins, Brittany 10
High-Maintenance Girl stereotype 51–52, 59–61, 67, 73–76
Hinge 16, 28
Hobbs, Mitchell 2
The Holiday 26
hook-up culture 3, 20, 28, 30–31, 84
Hoque, Anna 15–16

Illouz, Eva 64, 71
intimacy: additional social media to foster 43, 49, 85; animation and 42, 44, 49, 85; busy-ness and 49–50, 85–86; chemistry and 33–34, 85; cultural construction of 39, 71; difficulties in defining 38–39; digital data surveillance and 39; digital intimacy vs. 39–40, 49–50, 71, 83–84; feelings of intense digital 47–49; investment and 44–47, 84–86; jagged love cycle and 39–40, 50; need for face-to-face interaction and 40–41, 44, 85; profile movement and 42–43, 85; sense of self and 41–42; surface-level judgement and 43–44, 84–85; use of dating app and 7, 39–42, 84–85

Jagged Love concept: cyclical dating app behavior and 6–7, 31–34, 37, 83, 85, 89; FOMO (fear of missing out) and 6–7, 31, 34, 35, 83; gender scripts and 52, 65, 67–68; intimacy and 39–40, 50; meet-cute trope and 27; vs. Liquid Love concept 6, 21
James, Donna 5, 15
Jamieson, L. 32, 38, 40–41, 44, 47

JJJ (anecdote) 71–72
Jukane-Hobein, Iveta 47

Kanai, Akane 61, 63
kiss.com 3

Lean, Garth 5, 15
LGBTQ+ community 4–5, 26, 28, 56–57
Liquid Love concept: busy-ness and 34–35, 49, 83; gender scripts and 52; jagged love concept vs. 21, 37; as paradigm for dating apps 6, 20–21, 82–83
Locke, Ollie 18

Macleod, Caitlin 5, 25
MagicLab 17
match.com 3, 16
Mateen, Justin 16
McAlister, Jodi 4, 6, 21, 31
McArthur, Victoria 5, 25
McCosker, Anthony 11
McEwen, Caryn 60–61
McGlotten, Shaka 32, 38
McLaren, Angus 24
McRobbie, Angela 2, 59, 64, 74, 80, 87
media: coverage of increase in dating app usage 12–14; effect on public health of 11; gendered characterization of Tinder and Bumble and 15, 28; patriarchal reporting around dating apps 7, 9–12, 14
meet-cute romantic trope 26–28, 36, 80–81
methodology 4–5, 76–77
#metoo movement 10, 18
Murrie, Linzi 6, 53–54, 86

OkCupid 13
"the-one" trope 28–29, 36, 72
Owen, Stephen 2

personal ads 3
public relations language 39, 59–60, 64, 71–72, 75, 87
Pym, Tinonee 11

racism 51, 55–57, 68, 70, 75, 89
Rad, Sean 16–17
Reynolds, Linda 10
Rogers, Jack 18
romantic comedies 1, 20, 29, 36–37
romantic literature 1, 29
romantic masterplot(s): anxiety around milestones of 29–31, 74–75, 78–82, 88; celebrities and 71–72, 75, 81; COVID-19 and 2, 20, 74, 78, 80–82; dating apps and 20, 36–37, 80–82; dating app uses outside of 35–37; gender and 25; heteronormativity and 4–5; intimacy and 49; Jagged Love cycle and 31–34; meet-cute romantic trope 26–28, 80–81; "the-one" trope 28–29; role of hook-ups in 30–31, 84; social media expressions of 72–73; use of as response to anxiety 25–26
Rossiter, Penny 56
RSVP.com 3

Seidman, Elie 13, 22, 40
sexual assault 8–12
sexual harassment 16–17
Sexually Transmitted Diseases (STDs) 3
sexual scripting 6; *see also* gender scripts
sex work 70
Shumway, David 29, 81
significant-other label 23
Simon, William 6
Slow Love podcast 69–70
social media: authentication of users and 5, 26; intimacy and 43, 49, 85; relationship launches and 39, 71–72, 75; romantic scripts and 72–73
straight time 4–5, 25

Tan (app) 70
Tinder: about 16–17; association with heterosexual users 15; Bumble and 16, 28; COVID-19 and 12–14, 22; entanglement of digital and IRL worlds and 40; Facebook and 5; functionality of 18–19; gender and 5, 14–16, 26; geospatial matching and 3; inaccessibility of to outsiders 8, 11, 76; LGBTQ+ community and 5; predictions of 36; release of 3; reporting on sexual abuse and 9–12; sexual harassment suit and 16–17; use of in Australia 3; video chat and 13
toxic masculinity 58–59, 65, 87

United Nations (UN) 22, 78
unsolicited explicit imagery 18

Vincent, Louise 60–61

Ward, Russel 86–87
Winch, Alison 63
Wolfe Herd, Whitney 15–18

Zhang, Michael 70–71

Made in the USA
Monee, IL
13 September 2026

62978963R10063